CRASH COURSE
Nervous System

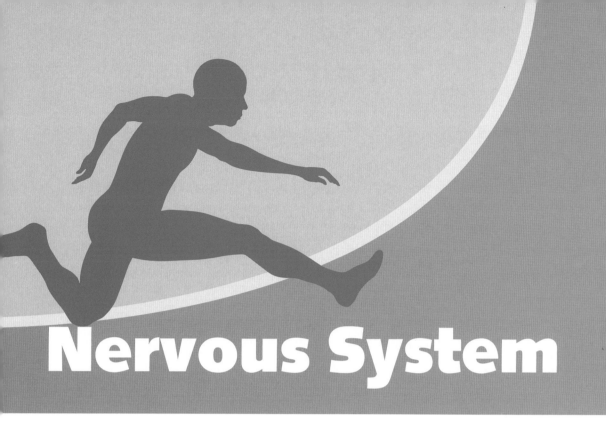

Nervous System

Gregory A. Mihailoff, PhD

Professor, Department of Anatomy and Neuroscience
Director, Office of Research and Sponsored Programs
Arizona College of Osteopathic Medicine
Glendale, Arizona

UK edition author
Charlie Briar

UK series editor
Dan Horton-Szar

ELSEVIER
MOSBY

**ELSEVIER
MOSBY**

1600 John F. Kennedy Blvd.
Ste 1800
Philadelphia, PA 19103-2899

CRASH COURSE: NERVOUS SYSTEM   ISBN 0-323-03443-8
Copyright 2005, Elsevier, Inc. All right reserved.

Previous editions copyrighted 1998, 2003.

Library of Congress Cataloging-in-Publication Data
Mihailoff, Gregory A.
 Nervous system / Gregory A. Mihailoff.
   p.   cm. — (Crash course)
 Rev. ed. of: Nervous system / Charlie Briar. London : Mosby, 2003.
 ISBN 0-323-03443-8
   1. Neurology—Outlines, syllabi, etc. 2. Nervous system—Outlines, syllabi, etc. I. Briar, Charlie. Nervous system. II. Title. III. Series.

RC357.B75   2005
612.8—dc22

                                                    2004065972

Commissioning Editor: Alex Stibbe
Project Development Manager: Stan Ward
Project Manager: David Saltzberg
Designer: Andy Chapman
Cover Design: Richard Tibbets
Illustration Manager: Mick Ruddy

Printed in China

Last digit is the print number: 9   8   7   6   5   4   3   2   1

Preface

Crash Course: Nervous System provides an integrated approach to the study of the nervous system. Combined in one text are fundamental anatomical and physiological concepts of systems neurobiology as well as basic topics in neuropathology and neuropharmacology. Also included are interesting clinical neurology topics that involve some of the more common presenting complaints in neurological disease and a section on the neurological exam. This edition concludes with a self-assessment chapter that contains multiple-choice and short-answer questions (and answers!).

The content of *Crash Course: Nervous System* makes it especially suitable for students who are beginning professional programs in medicine or allied health sciences. Second-year medical students preparing for national board exams will find this text useful as an integrated overview of basic and clinical neuroscience material. Residents in psychiatry, radiology, or internal medicine might also find this text useful because of the comprehensive review of a diverse array of topics involving the nervous system. This text will not serve as a detailed, in-depth reference source for topics in neuroscience, but it is my hope that its most redeeming feature is the wide breadth and broad scope of its treatment of basic and clinical neuroscience.

Greg Mihailoff, Ph.D.

Acknowledgments

As I look back in time, I realize how fortunate I have been to fall under the guidance of several very special individuals. Sincere thanks to Dr. James S. King and Dr. George F. Martin, Ohio State University College of Medicine for giving me the opportunity to evolve as a student of the nervous system in an excellent doctoral program. Dr. Rupert S. Billingham, University of Texas Southwestern Medical School, my first Chairman, proved to be an excellent role model for a young academician/research scientist. Many thanks to a friend and colleague, Dr. Duane Haines, University of Mississippi Medical Center, who, at mid-career, provided me with my first opportunity to participate in a major textbook project. And lastly, thanks very much to Dr. Ross Kosinski who was instrumental in recruiting me to my present position at Midwestern University even after he worked as a postdoctoral fellow in my laboratory for several years!

To my wife Rita and our three wonderful progeny, Kimberly, Mark and Laura, all of whom missed out on time with their husband/father when he was at the lab in those early days in Carrollton, Texas. I will never forget your sacrifices and any success I might achieve is your success.

Greg Mihailoff

Contents

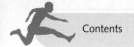

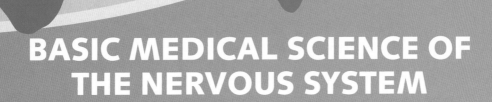

BASIC MEDICAL SCIENCE OF THE NERVOUS SYSTEM

1. Overview of the Nervous System

In this chapter, you will learn about:
- The anatomy of the central nervous system.
- The development of the central nervous system.
- The blood supply and venous drainage of the central nervous system, cerebrospinal fluid, and supporting cells of the central nervous system.

Introduction

The nervous system is divided into two anatomically different components. These are:
- Central nervous system, including all the structures contained within the cranium and spinal column.
- Peripheral nervous system, which contains the nerves and ganglia (groups of nerve cell bodies) outside the brain and spinal cord beginning with the anterior and posterior roots. The nervous system is further divided into somatic and autonomic branches:
  - The somatic portion contains the sensory and motor supply to skin, muscles, and joints.
  - The autonomic division supplies smooth muscle and glands along with some specialized structures, such as the pacemaker cells of the heart. One of its main functions is the control of the internal environment.

The nervous system is designed to detect features of the internal and external environments, to process this information, and to use it to direct behavior and body processes. There are three basic processes that work together to achieve this.

Perception

Specialized receptors in the skin respond to touch, pain, and temperature. Those in muscle respond to muscle length and others in joints respond to the position of the joint. These, together with information gathered by the special sense organs (for sight, hearing, balance, smell, and taste), provide the brain with information about the immediate and remote external environment and the body's position in space. There are also receptors which monitor the state of the internal environment (e.g., baroreceptors for blood pressure).

Information transfer and processing

Neurons (nerve cells) have specialized projections called axons that conduct trains of electrical impulses over long distances. The information delivered to neurons can be modified by, or integrated with, other inputs from related areas. In the central nervous system, neurons have many complex connections, allowing the brain to use the information in several different ways at once.

Output to body

Once the information has been collated and processed by the brain, it is then used to drive the output of the central nervous system. This includes supply to other excitable cells, such as muscles, internal organs, and glands (e.g., the diaphragm, heart, and hormone-producing centers such as the adrenals). In this way, the brain can control movement of the body and also modify the circulation and respiration.

Anatomy of the central nervous system

The fully developed central nervous system is shown in Fig. 1.1.

The cerebral cortex is divided into four lobes on the basis of the folds (sulci) in the surface, as shown in Fig. 1.2.
- The frontal lobe is separated from the parietal lobe by the central sulcus.
- The temporal lobe is separated from these by the lateral sulcus.
- Demarcation of the occipital lobe is difficult to appreciate from a lateral view but, on the medial (midsagittal) view (Fig. 1.3), the parieto-occipital sulcus can be seen quite clearly.

The paired lateral ventricles (Fig. 1.4) including the frontal, temporal, and occipital horns are

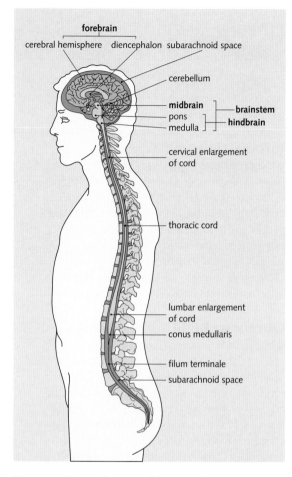

Fig. 1.1 Midsagittal section of the central nervous system showing components of the forebrain, midbrain, hindbrain, and spinal cord.

connected to the single (midline) third ventricle, which lies posterior and inferior, through the interventricular foramen of Monro. The third ventricle is joined to the fourth ventricle via the midline cerebral aqueduct (iter). The ventricles of the brain contain cerebrospinal fluid (CSF) and are joined together and to the subarachnoid space outside the brain and spinal cord to allow CSF to circulate around the brain.

The ventricles can sometimes be distorted by pressure exerted upon them by, for example, a tumor. Computed tomography and magnetic resonance imaging are useful studies to demonstrate this "mass effect."

Blood supply to the central nervous system

Fig. 1.5 shows the arteries which provide the blood supply to the brain. These form an anastomosis (different arteries supply blood to the same area), known as the Circle of Willis. Fig. 1.6 shows the territories of the major arteries supplying the cortex.

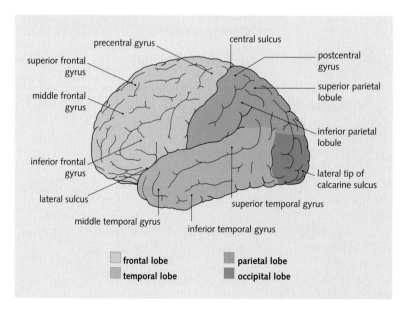

frontal lobe
temporal lobe
parietal lobe
occipital lobe

Fig. 1.2 Left cerebral hemisphere, lateral view showing major lobes.

Fig. 1.3 Medial view of the right side of the brain, showing deep structures, midbrain, and hindbrain.

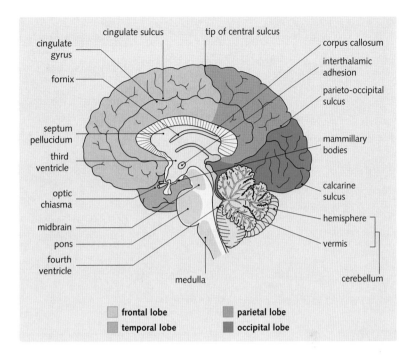

Fig. 1.4 The lateral ventricle, and its relationship to the basal ganglia and thalamus.

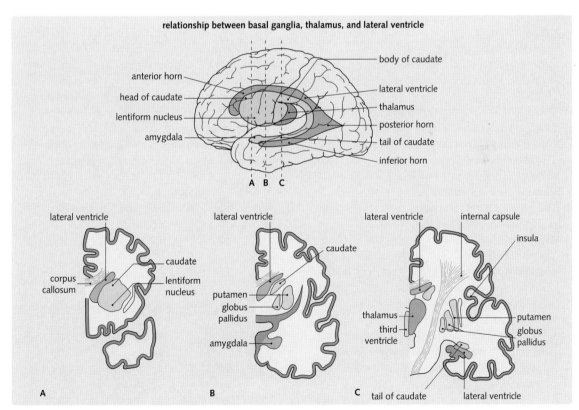

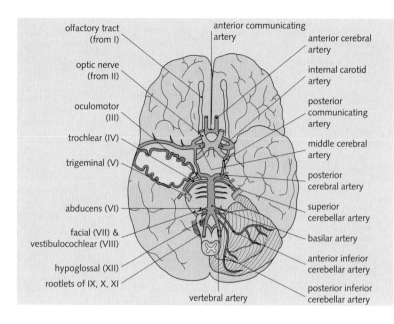

olfactory tract
(from I)

optic nerve
(from II)

oculomotor
(III)

trochlear (IV)

trigeminal (V)

abducens (VI)

facial (VII) &
vestibulocochlear (VIII)

hypoglossal (XII)

rootlets of IX, X, XI

vertebral artery

anterior communicating
artery

anterior cerebral
artery

internal carotid
artery

posterior
communicating
artery

middle cerebral
artery

posterior
cerebral artery

superior
cerebellar artery

basilar artery

anterior inferior
cerebellar artery

posterior inferior
cerebellar artery

Fig. 1.5 Blood supply to the brain, showing the Circle of Willis and its relationship to the cranial nerves.

A broad knowledge of these is helpful when assessing a person with a stroke.

Four vessels supply the brain—the right and left internal carotid arteries, and the paired vertebral arteries.

- The internal carotid artery sends off two branches (anterior and posterior communicating arteries) before continuing as the middle cerebral artery. This artery has an extensive territory, covering the majority of the lateral surface of the brain and also some of the basal ganglia.
- The anterior cerebral artery travels forward on either margin of the longitudinal fissure to supply the medial surface of each cerebral hemisphere.
- The vertebral arteries join at the inferior border of the pons to form the basilar artery. Branches of the vertebral arteries and the basilar artery supply the medulla, pons, and cerebellum.
- The paired posterior cerebral arteries, which supply the occipital and temporal lobes, derive from the basilar artery, with some contribution from the carotid vessels via the posterior communicating arteries.

The loop formed between the basilar artery and the internal carotid vessels via the anterior and posterior communicating arteries is known as the Circle of Willis.

The venous drainage of the cerebral cortex is funneled primarily into the superior sagittal sinus, which runs in the upper margin of the longitudinal fissure. This large sinus drains into the transverse sinuses where it joins blood from the cerebellum and brainstem (Fig. 1.7).

Optic, olfactory, and some facial structures drain into the cavernous sinus, which contains within its lumen or its walls many important structures, including:

- Internal carotid artery.
- Cranial nerves III, IV, VI, and the ophthalmic division of V.

Atherosclerosis in the common carotid artery or carotid bifurcation may cause blood clots to travel up the internal carotid artery. Due to the anatomy, it is most likely that the clot will travel to the middle cerebral artery territory and cause a stroke.

Fig. 1.6 Territories of the cerebral arteries. (A) Lateral and (B) medial views of the left and right cerebral hemispheres respectively. (C) Coronal (transverse) section of the cerebral hemispheres.

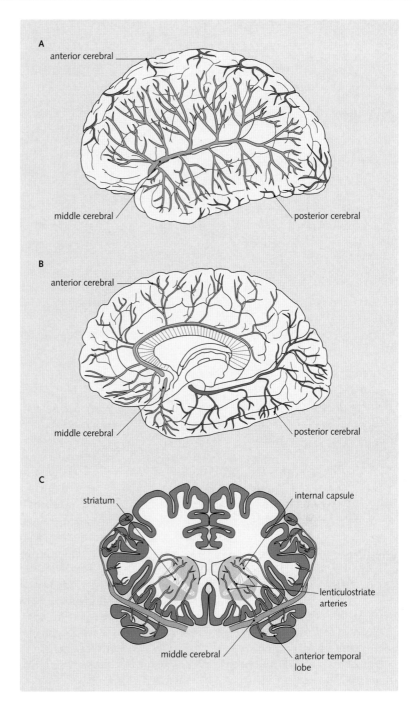

The cavernous sinus drains to the transverse sinus via the superior petrosal sinus and directly to the internal jugular vein via the inferior petrosal sinus.

The inferior sagittal sinus and the internal cerebral veins drain the deep structures of the cortex into the straight sinus, which empties into the confluence of sinuses and from here blood passes to the paired transverse sinuses, then to the paired sigmoid sinuses, and finally into the internal jugular veins which form at the jugular foramen.

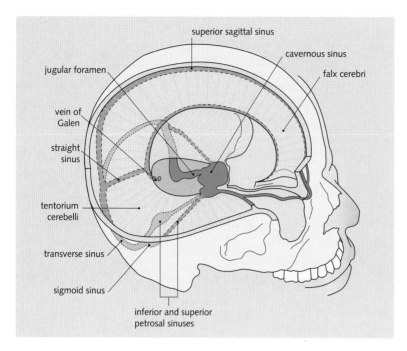

Fig. 1.7 The venous sinuses.

superior sagittal sinus

cavernous sinus

jugular foramen

falx cerebri

vein of Galen

straight sinus

tentorium cerebelli

transverse sinus

sigmoid sinus

inferior and superior petrosal sinuses

Spread of infection from the face or orbit may result in cavernous sinus thrombosis, producing a red swollen eye and palsies of the nerves running through it. On fundoscopy, papilledema may be seen.

Overall development of the nervous system

Development of the nervous system begins early in gestation, at approximately 3 weeks. There are three layers to the embryo at this stage:

- Endoderm (which forms the gastrointestinal tract and other internal organs).
- Mesoderm (which gives rise to muscles, connective tissue, and blood vessels).
- Ectoderm (which forms the nervous system and the skin).

Neurulation

At around day 22 of gestation, an area of ectoderm on the dorsal surface of the embryo, called the neural plate, thickens and folds to form the neural groove.

The ridges on either side of the groove expand and begin to fuse in the midline approximately halfway along its length (at the level of the 4th somite). Somites are paired blocks of mesoderm, segmentally arranged alongside the neural groove. The very tips of the ridges of the neural groove become the neural crest, and the fused neural tube gives rise to the brain and spinal cord. The tube at the cranial (rostral or head-end) neuropore fuses on day 25, and the caudal (or tail-end) neuropore on day 27. The stages of neurulation are shown in Fig. 1.8.

Neural crest cells migrate to form most of the cells in the peripheral nervous system, along with autonomic ganglia, cells of the adrenal medulla, and melanocytes in the skin.

By the end of development, the segmental arrangement of the nervous system determined by the somites is retained only in the spinal cord.

Embryology of the spinal cord

The neural tube is hollow, with the center becoming the spinal canal. Neuroblast cells, which surround the canal, divide and move outward from the center of the neural tube to ultimately form nerve cells and the gray matter of the spinal cord. These cells then send out nerve fibers that grow more peripherally into the marginal zone, and form the white matter of the spinal cord.

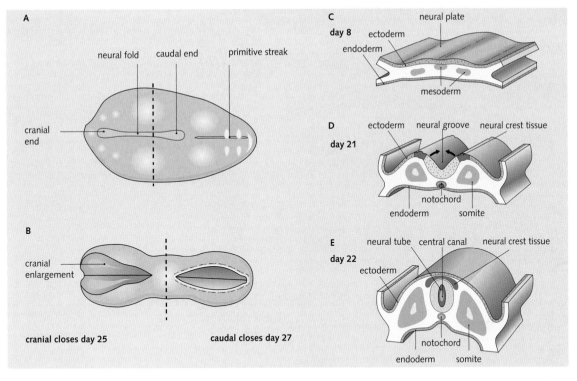

Fig. 1.8 Stages of neurulation. (A) Early embryonic disk. (B) Progression to formation of brain vesicles and spinal canal. (C–E) Transverse sections of neural tube taken at different stages of development.

If the cranial neuropore fails to close, the fatal condition of anencephaly results—the embryo continues to develop but the brain does not, and the structures that would normally overlie the brain are prevented from forming normally. This typically results in spontaneous abortion. Failure of the caudal neuropore to close results in disruption of the lumbar and sacral segments of the cord. Structures that lie superficial to the cord are also involved (e.g., meninges, vertebral arch, paravertebral muscles, and skin) because their development relies upon closure of the neural tube. Malformations involving the vertebral arch and the cord are called spina bifida.

The neuroblasts in the primitive gray matter form two populations—a dorsal alar plate and a ventral basal plate separated by a shallow groove (sulcus limitans).
- The alar plate cells form the sensory cells of the posterior (dorsal) horn.
- The basal plate cells form the motor cells of the anterior (ventral) horn along with sympathetic (in the thoracic region) and parasympathetic (in the lumbar and sacral regions) preganglionic neurons.

Fig. 1.9 shows the formation and development of the alar and basal plates.

Neural crest cells around the neural tube form the coverings of the brain and spinal cord:
- Pia mater (nearest the neural tube).
- Arachnoid mater.
- Dura mater (outer layer).

In the first 8 weeks of gestation, the spinal cord is the same length as the vertebral column. After this time,

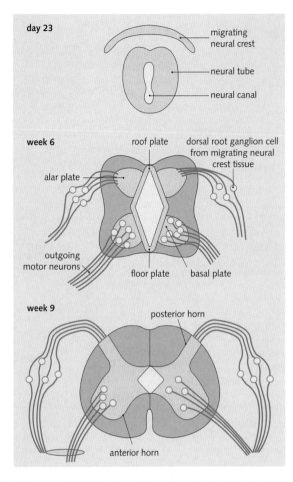

day 23

migrating neural crest

neural tube

neural canal

week 6

roof plate

dorsal root ganglion cell from migrating neural crest tissue

alar plate

outgoing motor neurons

floor plate

basal plate

week 9

posterior horn

anterior horn

Fig. 1.9 Cross-sections through the developing spinal cord, showing development of alar and basal plates and the primitive beginnings of inflow and outflow tracts.

Cauda equina syndrome. A prolapsed intervertebral disk or fracture can cause compression of the cauda equina. The symptoms of this include pain in the nerve distribution of the root affected, saddle anesthesia (around the anus), and disturbance of bladder/bowel function. It is a neurosurgical emergency and the pressure must be relieved to preserve the function of the nerves.

the vertebral column grows at a faster rate so that, by 40 weeks of gestation (term), the spinal cord stops at the level of L3 and, in adults, it ends at the L1/L2 disk space. The anterior and posterior roots (cauda equina) for those spinal nerves below this level in the adult descend within the subarachnoid space (lumbar cistern) until they reach the appropriate exit foramen. A thickening of the pia mater sweeps off the caudal tip of the spinal cord, the conus medullaris, and forms a round strand of tissue (filum terminale internus) that extends further caudally with the cauda equina to the termination of the dural sac at S2. External to the dural sac, a prolongation of the dura mater, the filum terminale externus continues to the region of the coccyx.

Embryology of the brain
General arrangement
The neural groove rostral to the 4th pair of somites enlarges before it fuses to form three primary brain vesicles or swellings.
- The tissue surrounding the first brain vesicle becomes the prosencephalon or forebrain.
- The tissue surrounding the second brain vesicle becomes the mesencephalon or midbrain.
- The tissue surrounding the third brain vesicle becomes the rhombencephalon or hindbrain.

Fig. 1.10 shows the fate of these vesicles.
Before the fifth week of gestation, the first and third vesicles each divide in two.
- The forebrain vesicle forms the telencephalon and diencephalon.
- The hindbrain vesicle forms the metencephalon and myelencephalon (or medulla).

The central canal of the neural tube enlarges to form:
- Lateral ventricles in the primitive cerebral hemispheres.
- Third ventricle in the diencephalon.
- Cerebral aqueduct (of Sylvius) in the midbrain.
- Fourth ventricle in the hindbrain.

The neural tube bends to form:
- The cervical flexure (between the primitive spinal cord and the third vesicle).
- The cephalic flexure (between the first and second vesicles).

10

Fig. 1.10 Development of the brain from the three-vesicle stage to adult areas.

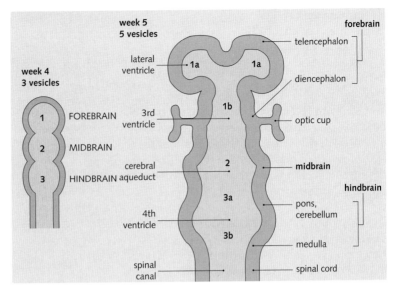

Development of the brainstem

The brainstem has the same basic structure as the spinal cord, except that it must accommodate the large motor and sensory tracts that run between the spinal cord and the brain.

Medulla

Initially, the myelencephalon or medulla is organized like the primitive spinal cord with alar and basal plates. As it flattens out more rostrally, forming the floor of the fourth ventricle, the alar plates (sensory cell groups) move outward until they lie lateral to the basal plates (motor cell groups). Other cells from the alar plate migrate ventrolaterally to form the olivary nuclei. This process is shown in Fig. 1.11.

The cells of the alar and basal plates are arranged in columns according to whether they innervate somatic (body wall) or visceral (internal organ) structures.

- The basal plate forms the motor nuclei for cranial nerves IX, X, XI, XII.
- The alar plate forms sensory nuclei for cranial nerves V, VIII, IX, X along with the gracile and cuneate nuclei (receiving inputs from the spinal cord).

Pons and cerebellum

The pons is formed by the anterior part of the metencephalon and part of the alar plate of the medulla. It contains a thick band of fibers (important in motor processing) which connect the forebrain with the cerebellum. The neurons of the ventromedial alar plate at this level form:

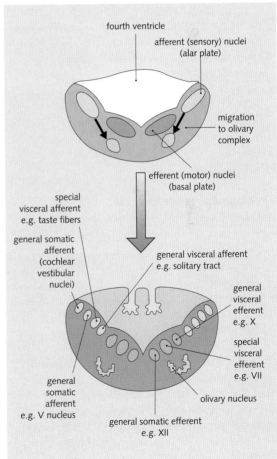

Fig. 1.11 Development of the medulla, with grouping of sensory and motor nuclei.

- The main sensory nucleus of V.
- A sensory nucleus of VII.
- Vestibular and cochlear nuclei of VIII.
- Pontine nuclei.

The neurons of the basal plate form the motor nuclei of V, VI, and VII. The cerebellum develops from the most posterior parts of the alar plates, rostral to the medulla. The cerebellar growths project over the top of the fourth ventricle and fuse in the midline, with the migrating cells from the alar plates becoming the cerebellar cortex.

Development of the midbrain
The midbrain retains the basic alar/basal plate structure. The neural canal becomes much narrower forming the aqueduct of the midbrain (also known as the aqueduct of Sylvius).
- The cells of the basal plate form the pure motor nuclei of the third and fourth cranial nerves, and possibly the red nucleus, substantia nigra, and reticular formation (involved in motor processing).
- The cells of the alar plates become the sensory neurons of the superior and inferior colliculi (involved in visual and auditory reflexes, respectively).

This is shown in Fig. 1.12.

Development of the forebrain
The part of the forebrain rostral to the optic vesicles becomes the telencephalon, containing:
- Cerebral cortex.
- Commisures (made up of corticocortical connections).
- Basal ganglia—which develop as swellings that protrude into the cavity of the lateral ventricles, along with the developing hippocampus.

The telencephalon (hemispheres) expands much more than the other parts of the brain, and ultimately covers the diencephalon and midbrain. The two swellings meet in the midline, trapping a small amount of mesenchymal tissue which forms the falx cerebri. The occipital lobes of the hemispheres similarly are separated from the cerebellum by mesenchyme, which becomes the tentorium cerebelli.

Grooves gradually appear on the smooth surface of the hemispheres, which become the sulci. The gyri

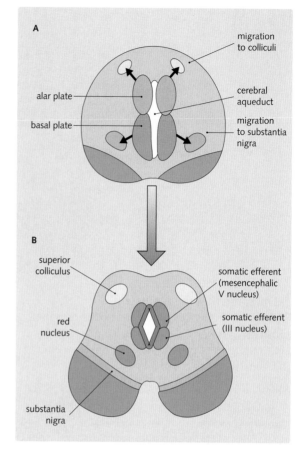

Fig. 1.12 Development of the midbrain, showing proximity to substantia nigra (basal ganglia).

thus formed allow a much greater volume of cortex (folded up) to be packed into the cranium. The cortex that covers part of the corpus striatum (lentiform nucleus) is called the insula. It remains fixed while the temporal, parietal, and frontal lobes rapidly grow to bury it within the lateral sulcus. This process is shown in Fig. 1.13.

The remainder of the forebrain becomes the diencephalon (Fig. 1.14), which contains:
- Hypothalamus (most rostral/ventral).
- The posterior pituitary gland and its stalk (the infundibulum).
- Thalamus.
- Epithalamus (most caudal/dorsal).

Pituitary gland
The pituitary gland is composed of two parts:
- A posterior (neural) part that develops from a downward growth (the infundibulum) from the floor of the hypothalamus.

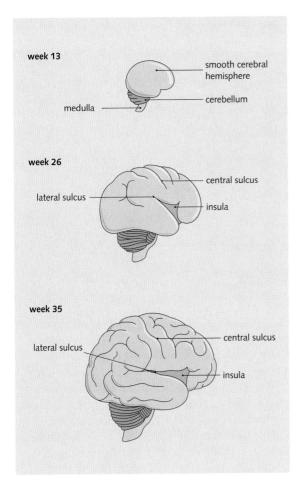

week 13

smooth cerebral hemisphere

cerebellum

medulla

week 26

central sulcus

lateral sulcus

insula

week 35

lateral sulcus

central sulcus

insula

Fig. 1.13 Growth of the cerebral cortex over the insula, and the development of gyri.

- An anterior (glandular) part that develops as an inward growth (Rathke's pouch) from the oral cavity toward the brain. It passes through the developing sphenoid bone to reach the downgrowth from the hypothalamus.

Development of the cranial nerves

There are three developmentally distinct groups of cranial nerves:

- Somatic efferents. These innervate muscles that develop from the parts of the rostral somites which become the head myotomes. This includes cranial nerves III, IV, VI to the ocular muscles, and XII to the tongue muscles.
- Pharyngeal arch nerves. These supply motor and sensory innervation to the embryological pharyngeal arches that formed the primitive oral cavity and pharynx. This group includes cranial nerves V (from the first arch), VII (second arch), IX (third arch), and X (fused fourth and sixth arches with the cranial branch of XI, the accessory nerve). The relationship of these nerves is shown in Fig. 1.15.
- Special sensory nerves. These afferent nerves relay information from special-sense receptors to the appropriate central pathway. This group includes cranial nerves I (olfaction), II (vision), and VIII (hearing and balance).

Development of the choroid plexuses

The choroid plexus is formed from two layers—the pia mater and the ependymal lining of the cavities of

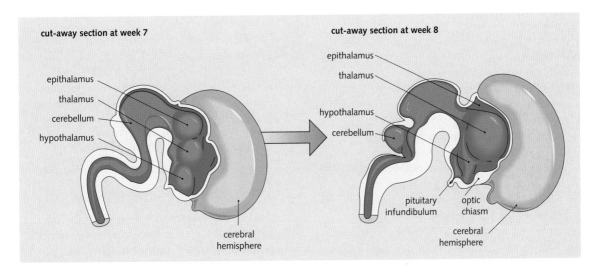

cut-away section at week 7

epithalamus
thalamus
cerebellum
hypothalamus

cerebral hemisphere

cut-away section at week 8

epithalamus
thalamus
hypothalamus
cerebellum

pituitary infundibulum
optic chiasm

cerebral hemisphere

Fig. 1.14 Development of the diencephalon showing cervical and cranial flexures.

13

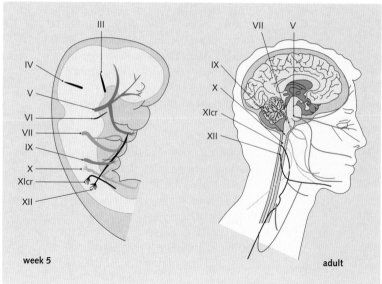

Fig. 1.15 Pharyngeal arch nerves in the embryo and adult.

the ventricles, which together are called the tela choroidea. This surrounds a core of vascular connective tissue that contains the blood supply. The tela choroidea push into the ventricles and develop into the choroid plexuses.

The central nervous system environment

Glial cells

Glial cells are the supporting cells for the neurons of the nervous system. Estimates suggest there are 5 to 10 times more glial cells than neurons in the nervous system.

Macroglia

- Schwann cell cytoplasm condenses into concentric lamellae around a single internodal segment on a single axon in the peripheral nervous system. This condensation of Schwann cell cytoplasm is called the myelin sheath.
- Oligodendrocytes are the equivalent of Schwann cells in the central nervous system, providing the myelin sheath. Unlike Schwann cells, each oligodendrocyte can myelinate many internodal segments on multiple axons.
- Astrocytes are small cells with long branching processes that provide the framework for the surrounding neurons (Fig. 1.16). They provide a kind of "scaffolding" which prevents axons of

different nerve cells from coming into contact with one another. Astrocytes also take up neurotransmitters, such as γ-aminobutyric acid (GABA) and glutamate, preventing them from constantly activating postsynaptic neurons. They store glycogen, which can be broken down to glucose in times of high metabolic demand, and help to regulate interstitial fluid potassium. They can replicate at sites of degeneration or traumatic injury and play a role in scar formation.

- Ependymal cells line the ventricles of the brain and the central canal of the spinal cord. Ependymocytes have cilia on their surface which project into the fluid-filled ventricular cavities and contribute to the flow of cerebrospinal fluid. They may also have a role in absorbing solutes from the cerebrospinal fluid.
- Choroidal epithelial cells are specialized ependymal cells that surround small arteries that protrude into the ventricular spaces and secrete cerebrospinal fluid.

Microglia

These cells are derived from macrophages outside the nervous system. Under normal circumstances, they appear to be inactive, but when there is tissue damage or inflammation they multiply and act as phagocytes. Similar to macrophages, they function as antigen-presenting cells and can therefore interact with other elements of the immune system.

Fig. 1.16 Glia, and their relationship to neurons and capillaries.

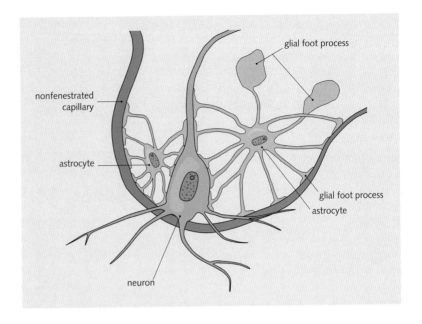

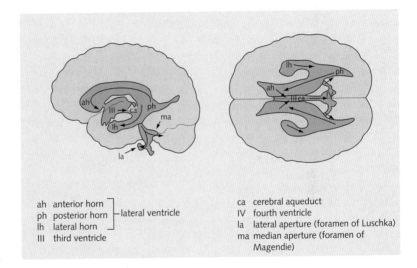

ah	anterior horn	
ph	posterior horn	lateral ventricle
lh	lateral horn	
III	third ventricle	

ca	cerebral aqueduct
IV	fourth ventricle
la	lateral aperture (foramen of Luschka)
ma	median aperture (foramen of Magendie)

Fig. 1.17 The ventricular system and the flow of cerebrospinal fluid.

Cerebrospinal fluid

Cerebrospinal fluid surrounds the brain and spinal cord (subarachnoid space) and is present in the ventricles and the central canal. It provides a cushion to prevent the delicate nervous tissue from being damaged. It also plays an active part in providing nutrition to the central nervous system, and removing waste products.

The majority of cerebrospinal fluid is formed by the choroid plexuses of the lateral, third, and fourth ventricles at the rate of about 500 mL/day. The total cerebrospinal fluid volume is approximately 150 mL, and this quantity must be turned over approximately three times a day. Groups of choroid plexus epithelial cells project into the ventricles, giving a folded appearance. These folds contain a leaky fenestrated capillary in the center, and on their surface have microvilli which project into the ventricles. The flow of cerebrospinal fluid is shown in Fig. 1.17.

Cerebrospinal fluid is produced by a combination of capillary filtration and active transport of solutes. Blood and cerebrospinal fluid are in osmotic equilibrium because water follows the gradients created. The differences between blood and cerebrospinal fluid are shown in Fig. 1.18. These

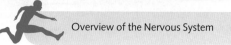

Fig. 1.18 The differences between blood and cerebrospinal fluid.

Differences between blood plasma and cerebrospinal fluid (CSF)		
	Plasma	CSF
Protein (mg/dL)	7000	35
Glucose (mg/dL)	90	60
Na (mmol/L)	138	138
K (mmol/L)	4.5	2.8
Osmolarity (mOsm/L)	295	295
pH	7.41	7.33

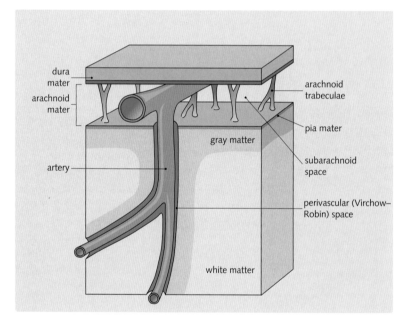

Fig. 1.19 Spaces filled with cerebrospinal fluid—subarachnoid and perivascular.

parameters can be measured by performing a lumbar puncture and obtaining a sample of cerebrospinal fluid.

Cerebrospinal fluid flows through the lateral and third ventricles into the cerebral aqueduct and eventually reaches the fourth ventricle. From there, it gains access to the subarachnoid space and the central canal of the spinal cord. The cerebrospinal fluid reaches the nervous tissue by traveling along blood vessels in the perivascular (Virchow–Robin) space (Fig. 1.19).

Cerebrospinal fluid is taken back into the venous circulation through arachnoid granulations (villi), which are formed by protrusions of the arachnoid membrane into the dural venous sinuses. The largest number of arachnoid villi are formed in the superior saggital sinus where the bulk of cerebrospinal fluid is absorbed into the venous circulation.

Lumbar puncture should not be performed on any individual who has elevated intracranial pressure because it may cause herniation of the cerebellar tonsils ("coning") and brainstem death—if in any doubt, a computed tomography head scan should be obtained first.

Hydrocephalus

This condition results from an increase in pressure within the ventricular system, usually due to a blockage in the flow of cerebrospinal fluid into the venous circulation. This is most likely to occur at the outlets from the fourth ventricle (the foramina of Luschka and Magendie), which are very narrow. It may also occur at the level of the cerebral aqueduct (of Sylvius). The latter condition is known as noncommunicating (or obstructive) hydrocephalus. Causes include:

- Tumors (either blocking flow of cerebrospinal fluid into the vascular compartment or producing excess cerebrospinal fluid).
- Congenital malformations of the brain and ventricular system.
- Infection (e.g., tuberculous meningitis) that obstructs the flow or resorption of cerebrospinal fluid.

Communicating hydrocephalus is caused by a blockage outside the ventricular system in the arachnoid space. This can be caused by:

- Meningitis.
- Subarachnoid hemorrhage.

The ventricles rostral to the blockage dilate and exert pressure on the surrounding brain tissue. This increases intracranial pressure and, especially in the newborn, can distort the skull bones (as the sutures have not fused at this stage).

The blood–brain barrier

The blood–brain barrier exists to maintain the environment of the brain in a steady state, protected from extracellular ion changes, peripheral hormones (such as adrenaline), drugs, and various other macromolecular substances. It also prevents neurotransmitters from entering the peripheral circulation (except in the pituitary gland and a few other locations, such as the circumventricular organs, where the blood–brain barrier is absent).

There are two factors that combine to maintain the balance between plasma and cerebrospinal fluid:

- The endothelial cells of the nonfenestrated cerebral capillaries have high resistance tight (occluding) junctions between them, and lack the methods of transcellular transport which are present in peripheral capillaries (fluid-phase and carrier-mediated endocytosis).
- Astrocytes have foot processes which adhere to the capillary endothelial cells (and are thought to help maintain the endothelial cell tight junctions). Thus the astrocytic foot processes play a role in the physiologial activity of the blood–brain barrier but do not participate in the actual physical barrier itself.

Small lipid-soluble molecules cross this barrier easily, but hydrophilic molecules must rely on specific transporter systems. D-Glucose, for example, has a stereospecific membrane transporter that facilitates diffusion from the circulation to the cerebrospinal fluid at high rates because the brain relies heavily on glucose for energy. However, in situations where there is a dramatic fall in plasma glucose levels (e.g., in diabetic hypoglycemic states), glucose may diffuse back out of the cerebrospinal fluid into the plasma. This is a medical emergency as the brain needs glucose to survive.

Other transport systems include those for amino acids—one each for basic (e.g., arginine), neutral (e.g., phenylalanine), and acidic (e.g., glutamate) amino acids. Clinically, the neutral transporter is important, as it will transport L-dopa (used as a treatment for Parkinson's disease, to replace dopamine lost from the substantia nigra). However, dopamine cannot be given as a treatment because it does not have a transporter and thus cannot cross the blood–brain barrier.

Abrupt changes in the ionic concentration can be damaging to neurons. The blood–brain barrier not only helps to protect the brain from such changes in plasma levels, but also helps to remove excess ions from the cerebrospinal fluid. For example, intense neuronal activity can increase the cerebrospinal fluid potassium concentration, and there is a high concentration of K^+ channels on endothelial cells which clear the excess.

Brain ischemia, brain tumors, hemorrhage, systemic acidosis, or infections such as bacterial meningitis may break down the blood–brain barrier.

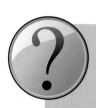 In diabetic ketoacidosis (where plasma glucose becomes excessively high), pH of the plasma may fall below 7, at which point the blood–brain barrier is compromised and neuronal death occurs.

Metabolic requirements of the central nervous system

The mechanisms within the blood–brain barrier provide the substrates for cellular metabolism in the brain via cerebrospinal fluid.

The brain is vulnerable to interruptions in its blood supply because it can store neither oxygen nor glucose, and cannot normally undergo anerobic metabolism. It has a high metabolic rate due to the energy demand of Na^+/K^+ ATPase pumps in the neuronal membranes. The brain consumes 20% of the body's oxygen and 60% of its glucose.

Under conditions of starvation for several days, the central nervous system can adapt to use ketones (fat derivatives acetoacetate and hydroxybutyrate) as its main energy source. These compounds normally make up approximately 30% of the fuel for the brain in adults but, after fasting for 40 days, this can rise to 70%.

- In infants, blood–brain barrier transport of glucose is 30% of the adult level, whereas ketone transport is approximately seven times as high. Amino acid transport in children is also higher than in adults, reflecting a higher rate of protein synthesis in the developing brain.

- What structures make up the brainstem?
- Describe the ventricular system within the brain.
- How is the neural tube formed? How might failure of fusion present?
- How does the diencephalon develop from the primitive forebrain?
- What are the functions of glial cells? How do macroglia and microglia differ?
- Explain the production and circulation of cerebrospinal fluid with reference to hydrocephalus.
- Compare the composition of plasma with that of cerebrospinal fluid.
- What is the blood–brain barrier? Why is it important?

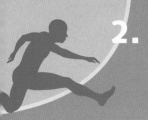

2. Cellular Physiology of the Nervous System

In this chapter, you will learn about:
- The structure of neurons and their networks.
- The action potential and transmission of impulses.
- Synaptic transmission.
- The effect of damage to the nervous system at the cellular level.

Neuronal structure and function

Introduction
The nervous system is highly complex, but the basic principles which underlie its function are fairly simple. Understanding these concepts is the first stage in appreciating the way in which the entire system functions.

Neurons
Neurons are excitable cells that are able to conduct electrical impulses and communicate with other excitable cells via specialized junctions called synapses. Although they vary considerably in their structure according to their location and function, a typical neuron is shown in Fig. 2.1.

> Certain viruses can exploit the retrograde transport of transmitter fragments from the axon to the cell body to gain access to the nervous system. These include the herpes simplex viruses, herpes zoster, rabies, and polio virus.

The cell body has a series of branching processes called dendrites which collect information from surrounding excitable cells and conduct it to the cell body. The number of dendrites in a cell reflects the way information is processed in that pathway. For example, a cell with many inputs may condense information from several pathways, whereas a cell with just a few few inputs may be part of a highly conserved parallel pathway.

The output of the nerve cell is a binary signal (meaning that it is an all-or-none impulse or train of impulses). The output is generated at the axon hillock when the cell's electrical threshold potential is reached. The output travels down another process extending from the cell body—the axon hillock and axon. In contrast to the dendrites, there is only one axon per neuron (although the axon may divide into numerous branches).

The axon transmits the output of the neuron (the action potential) to the terminal (synaptic) boutons, which are presynaptic swellings containing vesicles or packets of neurotransmitter. Different arrangements of the cell body and its processes are shown in Fig. 2.2.

Arrangement of neurons
According to their function, neurons can be arranged as:
- Layers (e.g., in the cerebral and cerebellar cortices) (Fig. 2.3).
- Rods or columns (e.g., motor neurons in the spinal cord).
- Nuclei (e.g., cranial nerve nuclei in the brainstem).

There are two classes of neuron:
- Projection neurons (called Golgi type-I neurons) influence cells located in a different part of the nervous system and so they tend to have relatively long axons (e.g., cortical motor neurons). The long axons often give off small collateral branches that help to spread information in the central nervous system. This type of neuron is distinct from projection neurons that have connections outside the nervous system. The latter neurons may be either afferent (or sensory) axons (e.g., from skin receptors) or efferent (motor) axons (e.g., to muscles or glands).
- Local interneurons (termed Golgi type-II neurons) have shorter axons that do not leave the nucleus where the cell body is located, and so provide opportunities for cells in that nucleus to communicate with each other. Often, the axons of these cells give off many collateral branches. This will increase the ability of the cells in the circuit to

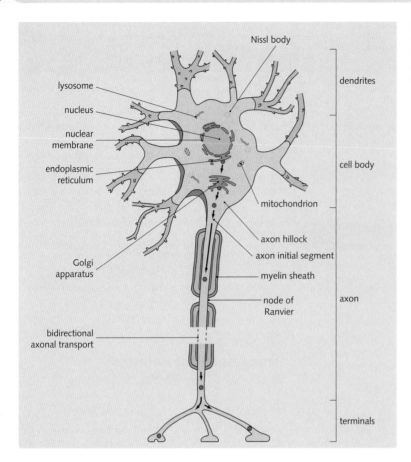

Fig. 2.1 Cellular features of a typical neuron. Note that although only anterograde transport is shown, retrograde movement of molecules also occurs.

process information. Humans have a much larger number of these types of neuron compared with their closest evolutionary relatives.

Neuronal excitation and inhibition

All nerve cells are electrically polarized (there is an electrical potential gradient across their membranes). The value of this potential determines whether a cell will or will not generate an action potential and it depends on the relative membrane permeabilities to the ions in the extracellular fluid (mainly Na^+ and Cl^-) and intracellular fluid (mainly K^+). The signal to alter permeability comes from neurotransmitter interaction with receptors at the synapse or direct electrical excitation of the neuron.

Similarly, the neuron may be inhibited from firing when the membrane potential is moved further away from the threshold value, typically by increasing its permeability to Cl^-.

Ionic basis of the resting potential

In the resting neuron, there is a great deal more potassium within the cell than outside, and much less sodium. The cell membrane is relatively impermeable to ions (although there is some outward leak of K^+). If there were no active channels at work, and no other ions were able to cross the membrane, then potassium ions would have a tendency to move out of the cell down their concentration gradient, leaving a relatively negative charge inside the cell. This would continue until the electrical force attracting the positive K^+ ions into the cell is equal (and opposite) to the chemical force of the concentration gradient. The electrical potential at which this equilibrium is reached for an ion is calculated by using the Nernst equation:

$$E_x \equiv \frac{RT}{zF} \ln \frac{[X_o]}{[X_i]}$$

where E_x is the equilibrium potential for ion X, R is the international gas constant, T is the temperature

Neurons can be demyelinated by diseases such as Guillain–Barré syndrome and multiple sclerosis. This causes slowing of conduction, and may even prevent axons from conducting impulses at all. Both conditions may result in paralysis or even death, although these changes are reversible in Guillain–Barré syndrome.

Synaptic transmission

Introduction

Synapses are junctions between the terminal bouton of the presynaptic neuron and its postsynaptic target cell (which may be another neuron, muscle, or gland cell). The junction comprises the membranes of both cells and a tiny gap between them, the synaptic cleft. Synapses alter the membrane potential of the postsynaptic cell and may be:

- Chemical (requires a neurotransmitter).
- Electrical (requires a cytoplasmic connection between the cells).

The differences between these types of synapses are shown in Fig. 2.7.

For chemically operated synapses (which make up the vast majority of junctions in the nervous system), the postsynaptic site contains specific receptor proteins that bind the released chemical neurotransmitter agent. This is essential for amplifying the signal from the neuron, as the extracellular current generated in the presynaptic neuron is not sufficient to cause a significant depolarization of the postsynaptic cell.

Types and location of synapses

Synapses (Fig. 2.8) may be:

- Excitatory (depolarizing—increasing the membrane permeability to Na^+ ($E_x = +55\,mV$) and thus moving the membrane potential of the postsynaptic cell toward its threshold level).
- Inhibitory (hyperpolarizing—increasing the membrane permeability to Cl^- ($E_x = -65\,mV$) or K^+ ($E_x = -75\,mV$), thereby moving the membrane potential of the postsynaptic cell further from its threshold).

The location of a synapse can enhance its action—the closer a synapse to the axon hillock of the postsynaptic cell, the greater its effect will be.

The most common sites for synapses are:

- Axodendritic. These comprise the most common form of synapse between neurons.
- Axosomatic. These are usually inhibitory, and when placed close to the axon hillock will more effectively inhibit postsynaptic cell firing than an axodendritic synapse since this is the site of action potential generation.
- Axoaxonic synapses. These can affect (modulate downward) the release of transmitter from the postsynaptic cell.

Process of transmission

Fig. 2.9 shows the steps between arrival of the action potential, transmitter release, and termination of transmitter effect.

Step 1: Action potential arrives at the terminal bouton and the depolarization opens voltage-gated calcium channels.

Comparison of electrical and chemical synapses		
Feature	Electrical	Chemical
cytoplasmic continuity	yes	no
delay	none	0.8–1.5 ms
agent	ion	neurotransmitter
space between cells	2 nm	30–50 nm
direction of signal	one way or both ways	one way
variation in function	either on or off	modifiable activity levels

Fig. 2.7 Comparison of electrical and chemical synapses.

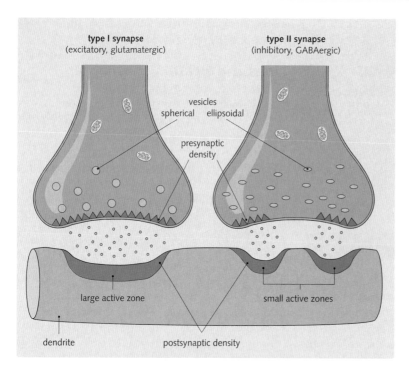

Fig. 2.8 Excitatory (depolarizing) synapse and inhibitory (hyperpolarizing) synapse.

type I synapse
(excitatory, glutamatergic)

type II synapse
(inhibitory, GABAergic)

vesicles
spherical   ellipsoidal

presynaptic
density

large active zone

small active zones

dendrite

postsynaptic density

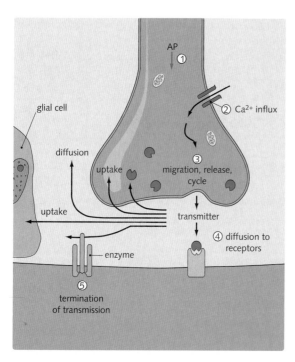

AP
①

glial cell

② Ca²⁺ influx

diffusion

uptake

③
migration, release,
cycle

uptake

transmitter

④ diffusion to
receptors

enzyme

⑤
termination
of transmission

Fig. 2.9 Synaptic transmission.

Step 2: Calcium ions enter the terminal bouton and allow the vesicles to attach to presynaptic release sites.

Step 3: The vesicle membrane fuses with the presynaptic membrane and the contents are released into the synaptic cleft. The vesicle membrane is then incorporated back into the membrane of the presynaptic terminal (recycled) to form more vesicles which are filled with transmitter for reuse. This is a potentially deleterious process because it allows extracellular contents to gain access to the interior of the nerve cell (e.g., polio virus or herpes virus).

Step 4: The transmitter diffuses across the synaptic cleft and binds to receptors on the postsynaptic membrane and, in some systems, to presynaptic receptors to regulate transmitter release.

Once the transmitter has bound to its postsynaptic receptors it causes a change in the postsynaptic membrane potential (either an excitatory or inhibitory postsynaptic potential, EPSP or IPSP). The size of this postsynaptic potential change is directly proportional to the number of vesicles released. If many vesicles are released, the resulting EPSPs are summed, and may cause the postsynaptic membrane potential to exceed the postsynaptic cell's threshold. The theory which correlates the number of EPSPs with the number of vesicles released is known as the quantum hypothesis (the amount of transmitter in each vesicle being a quantum). The effects of EPSPs and IPSPs on the membrane potential are shown in Fig. 2.10.

The effect of the chemical transmitter is terminated (Step 5) by one or more of the following mechanisms:

- Enzymatic degradation of the transmitter in the cleft (e.g., acetylcholinesterase in cholinergic neurons).
- Reuptake of the transmitter into the terminal bouton.
- Uptake of transmitter into glial cells.
- Diffusion out of the cleft.

Modulation of these mechanisms forms an important basis for central nervous system therapeutic intervention.

Temporal and spatial summation

Temporal summation occurs when a number of action potentials arrive at intervals that are shorter than the EPSPs they evoke. These EPSPs then summate (add together) to move the membrane potential of the postsynaptic neuron above threshold. These EPSPs must occur very close in time since the individual membrane fluctuations they cause will decay after a relatively short time. Spatial summation occurs when a number of different synapses located on the same neuron all evoke EPSPs at approximately the same time. Again, all the EPSPs add together to move the membrane potential above

threshold. Fig. 2.11 shows the difference between temporal and spatial summation. The same principles apply to IPSPs, except that the membrane potential moves away from its threshold level.

Facilitation

If a number of action potentials reach a terminal bouton in a short space of time, then gradually the effect of the transmitter on the postsynaptic cell is enhanced (i.e., either more excitation or more inhibition occurs). This may be due to a buildup of Ca^{2+} within the presynaptic bouton causing increased exocytosis as a result of increased Ca^{2+} entry outstripping the removal mechanism. Facilitation can only be sustained as long as there is transmitter in the vesicles. The enzymes that generate transmitter molecules and peptide transmitters are synthesized in the cell body and transported along the axon, which takes time. The facilitatory effect is therefore not sustained indefinitely.

Neurotransmitters and their receptors

There are five major types of neurotransmitter. An example of the synthesis of each is given in Fig. 2.12:

- Acetylcholine. This is the transmitter at the neuromuscular junction (NMJ) and also at many points in the autonomic nervous system. The cholinergic pathways in the brain may be important for memory formation, as anticholinesterase drugs seem to help people with Alzheimer's disease and anticholinergics make their symptoms worse.

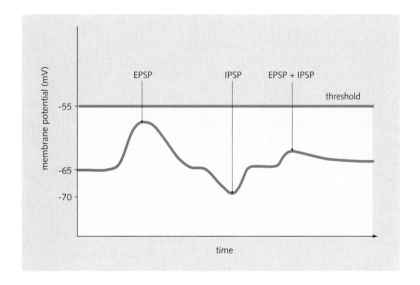

Fig. 2.10 Effects of excitatory postsynaptic potential (EPSP) and inhibitory postsynaptic potential (IPSP) on the membrane potential.

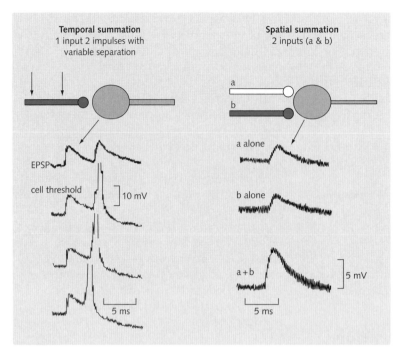

Fig. 2.11 Temporal and spatial summation.

- Amines (dopamine, noradrenaline, 5-hydroxytryptamine). The central pathways of the neurons containing these transmitters come mainly from the brainstem, and they have important actions on all parts of the brain. The monoamine pathways are often modified when treating people with depression, but it is not known exactly how the drugs work.
- Excitatory amino acids (glutamate, aspartate). Glutamate is the most important excitatory amino acid, and is extremely widespread throughout the central nervous system. There are two main classes of glutamate receptors: the AMPA receptor and the NMDA receptor. The latter is thought to be an important component in long-term potentiation and in memory formation. Glutamate is highly toxic to the brain in large quantities, possibly mediated by Ca^{2+} influx through the NMDA receptors, which are widespread throughout the cortex. This may be the cause of neuronal cell death in status epilepticus.
- Inhibitory amino acids (GABA, glycine). GABA is a derivative of glutamate and is widespread throughout the central nervous system, whereas most of the glycine-containing cells are interneurons in the spinal cord. Both are thought to cause hyperpolarization via the influx of Cl^-

ions thereby taking the neuron further away from its threshold potential.
- Peptides (opioids, neuropeptide-Y, substance-P, somatostatin). This is an extremely diverse group, with equally wide-ranging functions. Some have hormone activity (somatostatin, insulin), others modulate nociceptive pathways in the spinal cord and brainstem (opioids). They are commonly released along with small molecules which themselves have neurotransmitter-like actions (e.g., ATP).

Myasthenia gravis is a condition caused by the formation of antibodies to the postsynaptic acetylcholine receptor. It is characterized by muscle weakness which becomes progressively worse with exercise. This is known as fatiguability. Diagnosis is made by observing an improvement in the symptoms (an increase in muscle strength) when a short-acting anticholinesterase (the tensilon test) is administered intravenously.

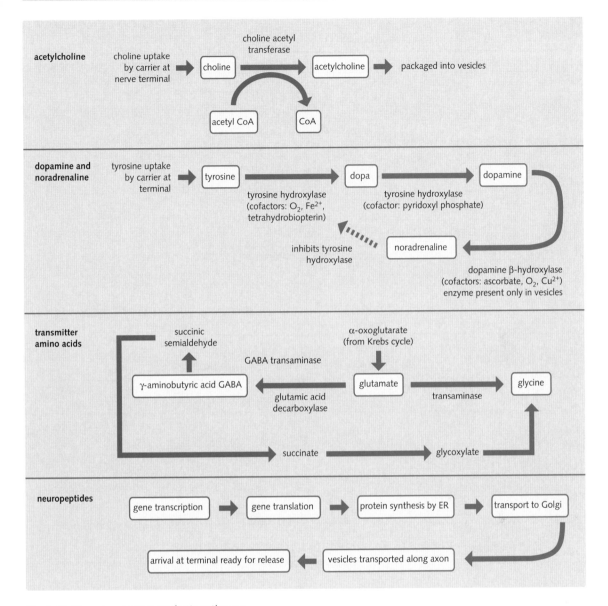

Fig. 2.12 Neurotransmitter synthetic pathways.

The effect of a neurotransmitter depends upon the type of receptor present at the synapse. Thus, one neurotransmitter can have different effects throughout the central nervous system, depending on which of its receptors is present there. Receptors can be classified according to the second messenger system that they use to alter the membrane potential. Two main classes of receptor are outlined in Fig. 2.13:

- The ionotropic receptor that is coupled with an ion channel for cations or anions. When these receptors are simulated, they have a direct effect on membrane potential.
- The metabotropic receptor that is coupled to a G-protein and uses cAMP (cyclic adenosine monophosphate) or IP$_3$ (inositol 1,4,5-triphosphate) as second messengers that can then have intracellular effects to bring about changes in ion channels to alter the membrane potential.

Receptor diversity for the major neurotransmitters is shown in Fig. 2.14.

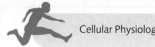

Structure and function of two main classes of receptor		
	Ionotropic	Metabotropic
structure	transmembrane ion channel composed of five subunits; binding sites for ligand and modulators outside cell	single transmembrane protein with sites for interaction with ligand outside cell and interaction with G-protein inside cell
functional units	each subunit has four transmembrane domains, and subunits create a charge field to attract either cations or anions; e.g., AChα subunit attracts Na$^+$, GABA$_B$ subunit attracts Cl$^-$	seven transmembrane domains with specific amino-acid residues within domains important for ligand binding; e.g., D$_1$ receptor has aspartate in domain 3 for dopamine binding

Fig. 2.13 Comparison between the two main types of neurotransmitter receptor—ionotropic and metabotropic.

Receptor diversity for the major neurotransmitters					
Transmitter	Cation channel	Anion channel	Increased cAMP by G-protein	Decreased cAMP by G-protein	Increased IP$_3$ by G-protein
ACh	nicotinic			M$_2$, M$_4$	M$_1$, M$_3$
dopamine			D$_1$	D$_2$	
glutamate (channels classified according to experimental agonists)	NMDA (Na$^+$, K$^+$, Ca^{2+}), kainate,and AMPA (Na$^+$, K$^+$)			mGluR2	mGluR1
GABA		GABA$_A$(Cl$^-$)		GABA$_B$	
opioids				μ, δ	

Fig. 2.14 Receptor diversity for the major neurotransmitters.

Regulation of transmitter synthesis

Transmitter synthesis can be regulated in the short term at the terminal bouton by the intracellular calcium level. If the neuron fires many action potentials, Ca^{2+} will build up at the terminal boutons and increase the activity of Ca^{2+}-dependent protein kinases which then influence the enzymes in the transmitter pathway. In the longer term, regulation occurs by second messenger actions on gene transcription of the rate-limiting enzyme. Fig. 2.15 shows these processes for dopamine regulation.

Neural networks

Different types of processing require different arrangements of connections in a neuronal circuit. Neurons that form the output from a particular circuit integrate information from that circuit and send it elsewhere. An extreme example is the cortical motor neuron that sends its axon in the corticospinal tract. A large number of neuronal contacts converge on the cell, because a number of different circuits govern voluntary movement. This is an example of convergence.

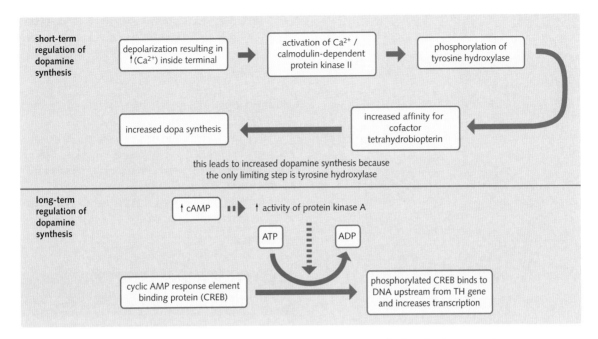

Fig. 2.15 Short- and long-term regulation of dopamine synthesis (TH, tyrosine hydroxylase).

Sensory information coming into the brain needs to go to different areas for processing. Pain, for example, has components of localization, intensity, and emotion, yet only a few receptors send this information to the central nervous system. The neurons in this circuit show a diverging pattern of connections such that similar information can be sent to different areas that are responsible for different aspects of pain perception. Visual information is initially kept separate as it is processed in the central nervous system in parallel pathways. This means that when certain neuronal groups are active, the brain appreciates that information is coming in from a restricted part of three-dimensional space and this increases our perceptual ability. At higher levels, this information is much more integrated so that we consciously perceive a picture rather than a collection of lines and colors in different areas of the visual field. At the cellular level, various arrangements of inhibitory connections can reduce "noise." Noise is background neuronal activity that is not connected with information carried in the circuit (i.e., noise makes the information in a circuit less clear). There are many patterns of inhibition with different functions:

- Recurrent inhibition is shown in Fig. 2.16. It permits a stable discharge without sudden surges in activity which could be deleterious. An example is seen in the spinal cord where spinal motor neurons are prevented from firing too often through connections with Renshaw cells. The most active cells activate the Renshaw cells maximally, thereby causing a global inhibitory feedback onto the group of related cells. In this way, only the most stimulated cells continue to fire, and the output of the group of cells becomes more focused.
- Lateral inhibition is shown in Fig. 2.17. Inhibitory interneurons can be used to "sharpen" a response, to give a distinct border between the "on" and "off" part of a receptive field.
- Presynaptic inhibition is shown in Fig. 2.18. An inhibitory synapse placed on a terminal bouton can reduce the membrane depolarization caused by an incoming action potential, probably by increasing the permeability to Cl^- so that when the interior of the cell becomes more positive with Na^+ current, Cl^- starts to move into the bouton. This will reduce the inward flow of Ca^{2+} and therefore also reduce transmitter release.
- Signaling by disinhibition also occurs. A cell at the end of a chain of neurons can be excited by inhibiting an inhibitory neuron earlier in the chain.

31

allow different kinds of processing to occur along the pathways (e.g., in relay nuclei), or may simply be an example of redundancy (useful if one pathway is damaged).

Connections

Commissural fibers connect neurons in different hemispheres. Association fibers connect neurons in the same hemisphere. There are vast numbers of connections in the central nervous system and there are many inputs modulating the effects of all connections. This means that even the simple reflex is influenced by other circuits and is not that "simple."

Damage and repair in the nervous system

A damaged axon will not conduct action potentials to its terminal boutons. This conduction block usually occurs either after section of the axon or demyelination of the axon.

The effect of demyelination

In myelinated axons, sodium channels are only present at the nodal regions, with the rest of the axon being electrically insulated. Fig. 2.19 shows that if myelin is removed, the current density at the nodal regions will be reduced because current will escape across the bare membrane.

A decrease in current density will depolarize the nodal region more slowly than normal, resulting in reduced conduction velocity. Because normal activation of the target site depends upon the timing as well as the number of action potentials in a population of fibers, any disruption in timing will lead to disruption of function. If more than one internodal segment is demyelinated, the severe decrease in longitudinal current may cause the current to fade along the length of the axon as more and more is lost across the membrane. This will prevent the axon from depolarizing to its threshold level, leading to conduction block. Fig. 2.20 shows how demyelination of axons in the central nervous system explains the clinical features of multiple sclerosis, where myelin sheaths are destroyed. The mechanism remains unknown but it may be due to an immune-mediated attack or an infection with an obscure pathogen.

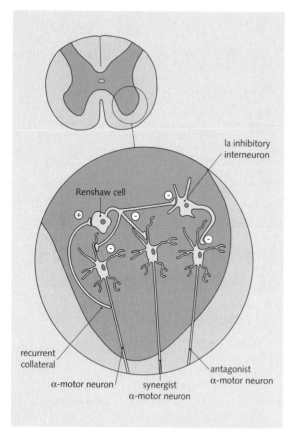

Fig. 2.16 Recurrent inhibition. When the alpha motor neuron is activated, it also activates the Renshaw cell, which in turn inhibits the motor neuron and synergistic motor neurons. It also relieves antagonistic motor neurons of their inhibition.

Inhibition is used in the creation of receptive fields, as shown in Fig. 2.17. A receptive field is the area which, when stimulated, causes a particular neuron to fire. It can be altered by inhibitory connections with neighboring sensory units. This can produce a receptive field where the receptor responds to stimulation in one area but is inhibited by stimulation immediately around that area, a so-called "on" center and an "off" surround (e.g., in retinal ganglion cells).

Looking at a higher level, there are connections between large groups of cells. Feedback loops between circuits encourage stable patterns of firing within individual circuits. Parallel pathways occur where there is more than one route that leads between two groups of cells. This arrangement may

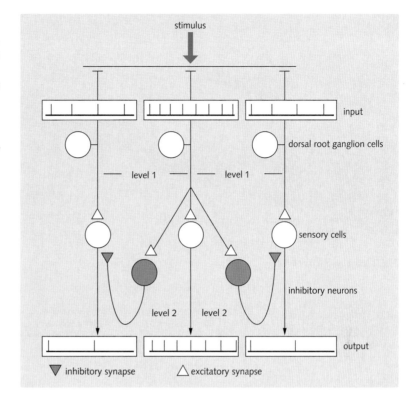

Fig. 2.17 Lateral inhibition. A stimulus causes a response in one receptor maximally and, to a lesser extent, in neighboring receptors. If solely excitatory neurons link the inputs (level 1), the signal becomes blurred. However, if inhibitory interneurons are introduced, then the cells which are not maximally stimulated will cease to fire. This sharpens the border between "off" and "on" (level 2) in a receptive field.

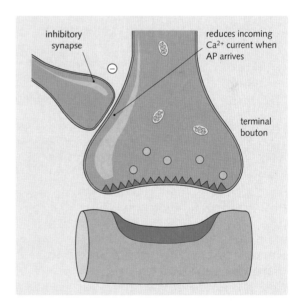

Fig. 2.18 Presynaptic inhibition preventing vesicle mobilization and release by decreasing calcium influx.

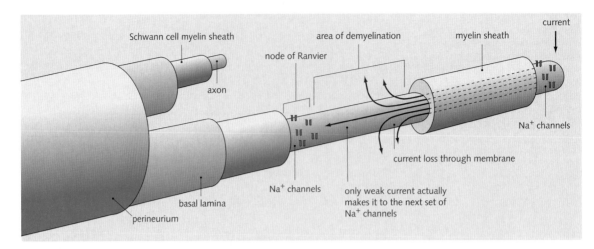

Fig. 2.19 The effect of demyelination on current flow in an axon.

Pathophysiology of multiple sclerosis symptoms	
Symptoms	**Cellular explanation**
blindness, numbness, weakness, paralysis	Block in conduction of action potential caused by dissipation of current after demyelination
paraesthesia (tingling)	Extracellular potassium builds up at sites of demyelination as channels exposed that leak potassium. This raises membrane potential to threshold and action potential generated spontaneously (Nernst equation)
remission of symptoms	Caused by: (A) remyelination by oligodendrocytes (B) use of alternative neural pathways (C) new sodium channels produced
relapse	(A) extension of existing lesion with exposure of membrane with few sodium channels (B) new lesion site
Lhermitte's sign (feeling of electric shock in limbs upon stretching)	Lesions often form in areas of CNS that are constantly being moved, such as the part of the spinal cord in the region of the cervical vertebrae. When lesioned axons are stretched they generate impulses. (A similar problem occurs in the optic nerve and flashes are seen at night when there is much less light to mask the effect of these spontaneous impulses.)

Fig. 2.20 Pathophysiology of multiple sclerosis symptoms.

Responses of peripheral axons to different types of trauma

Fig. 2.19 shows the relationship between a peripheral axon, its associated Schwann cells and thin connective-tissue covering—the basal lamina—which forms a continuous tube containing the axon–Schwann cells complex.

Fig. 2.21 shows that, after trauma, the main factors influencing restoration of function are the integrity of the axon itself, the integrity of the basal lamina, and the length of time needed for regrowth to the site of innervation (i.e., distal muscles may atrophy completely before a nerve sectioned far away grows and reaches them).

Responses of the central nervous system to damage

The central nervous system is hostile to axonal regrowth. Neurons will not grow through glial scars, and inhibitory molecules, associated with

Effects of peripheral nerve injury				
	Compression	Crush	Severed nerve	Severed limb
axon	intact	discontinuous	discontinuous	discontinuous
basal lamina	intact	intact	discontinuous	discontinuous
regrowth possibilities	no regrowth needed, full remyelination within a few weeks	trophic factors released by distal part of axon, and proximal axon (still attached cell body) regrows at 1 mm/day	trophic factors released by distal part of axon, but can grow into wrong basal lamina, previously occupied by nerve with different function	no distal part of axon present; nerve forms a neuroma
restoration of function	complete	dependent on length of axonal growth needed for reinnervation	four possibilities: 1. grows into original basal lamina 2. grows into basal lamina of same modality—altered function 3. grows into basal lamina of different modality—no function 4. forms neuroma—no function	no function; disturbed sensation and chronic/transient pain

Fig. 2.21 Effects of peripheral nerve injury.

oligodendrocytes, lead to failure of remyelination and cause a collapse of the growing tip of the axon. It is possible that cells secreting antibodies to the inhibitory molecules could be inserted locally in the tissue protecting the growth cone from inhibitory signals. Alternatively, in the case of spinal-cord injury, a piece of peripheral nerve could be inserted above and below the transection to provide a growth-friendly bridge across the gap.

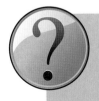

- Describe the basic structure of a neuron and comment on the function of the individual elements.
- What is the difference, anatomically and functionally, between projection neurons and interneurons?
- What is meant by the "resting potential" of a cell, and how is it maintained?
- Describe the sequence of events involved in an action potential.
- How is an action potential propagated along an axon?
- How do electrical and chemical synapses differ?
- What is the series of steps involved in chemical synaptic transmission starting from the action potential arriving at the terminal bouton?
- Explain the difference between temporal and spatial summation.
- What patterns of inhibition do you know? Describe them.
- What is the effect of demyelination on the conduction of action potentials?
- Name the common types of peripheral nerve function and the cellular processes of repair which allow restoration of function.

3. The Spinal Cord

In this chapter, you will learn about:
- The anatomy of the spinal cord.
- The tracts within the cord, and the modalities they subserve.
- The effect of damage to the spinal cord.

The spinal cord

The spinal cord is a segmentally organized tube with a central cellular area surrounded by nerve-fiber tracts. The tracts carry information between different levels of the spinal cord, and also to and from the supraspinal structures.

Fig. 3.1 shows the relationship between the spinal cord, its coverings, and its bony housing in the vertebral column. In adults, the cord ends at vertebral disk level L1/L2 and so a lumbar puncture needle can be inserted into the subarachnoid space below this level (e.g., L3/L4) without damaging the cord.

The presence of oligoclonal bands of protein in the cerebrospinal fluid on electrophoresis suggests the presence of large quantities of immunoglobulins. This is a feature of multiple sclerosis.

Cells

Fig. 3.2 shows that the cells in the central gray matter can be divided up as a series of layers in the dorsal horn and as a series of columns in the ventral horn. These layers and columns are known as Rexed's laminae (numbered I–X) and are based on groupings of similarly shaped cell bodies.
- The dorsal horn layers are involved in sensory pathways and are the target sites for some sensory afferent nerves, particularly for pain, temperature, and crude touch.
- The ventral columns are made up of pools of motor neurons innervating skeletal muscle. Medial motor columns supply proximal muscles and lateral motor columns supply distal muscles.
- In between the dorsal and ventral horns lies the interomediolateral column where the cell bodies of preganglionic sympathetic neurons are found.

The spinal tracts

As a general rule, in the white matter, the ascending sensory tracts run in the periphery and descending motor tracts occupy a more central position, as shown in Fig. 3.3. Sensory inputs from the skin terminate in laminae I–IV, with some fibers traveling to the segments above and below in Lissauer's tract.

Ascending pathways
The major difference between the main sensory tracts is that fine touch information (dorsal column tract) is conveyed up the cord on the same side as it enters, whereas pain, temperature, and crude touch (spinothalamic tract) are conveyed upward on the opposite side of the cord. The point at which the tract crosses to the contralateral side is known as the decussation.

The sensory tracts are both arranged segmentally (i.e., fibers from the same level run upward together in the tract). At the top of the dorsal columns, the segments are arranged in a coherent pattern from medial (sacral) to lateral (cervical), maintaining the body pattern. The pattern is distorted by divergence and convergence in the dorsal column nuclei so that distal structures (such as the hands) have a greater representation.

The dorsal column pathway
One of the functions of this pathway is to rearrange the input from the dermatomal input of the primary sensory fibers into the grossly distorted map of the body surface seen in the primary sensory cortex (the sensory homunculus). Here, the body surface is seen as grossly distorted with most of the cortical cells responding to sensory exploratory structures such as the hands, feet, and lips.

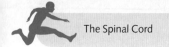

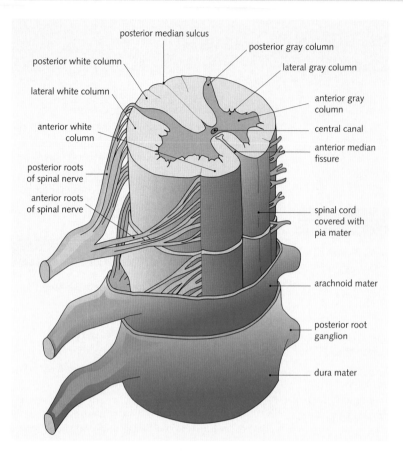

Fig. 3.1 Spinal cord above the level of L1, showing the meningeal coverings (dura mater, arachnoid mater, and pia mater).

posterior median sulcus

posterior gray column

posterior white column

lateral gray column

lateral white column

anterior gray column

anterior white column

central canal

anterior median fissure

posterior roots of spinal nerve

anterior roots of spinal nerve

spinal cord covered with pia mater

arachnoid mater

posterior root ganglion

dura mater

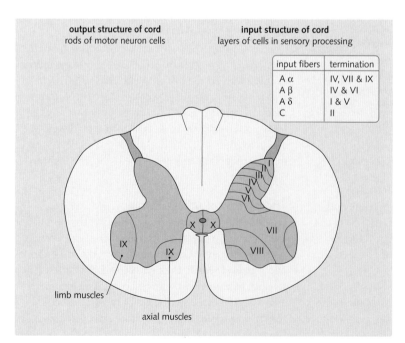

output structure of cord
rods of motor neuron cells

input structure of cord
layers of cells in sensory processing

input fibers	termination
A α	IV, VII & IX
A β	IV & VI
A δ	I & V
C	II

limb muscles

axial muscles

Fig. 3.2 Rexed's laminae. The different termination patterns of afferent fibers are shown.

Fig. 3.3 Ascending and descending spinal tracts.

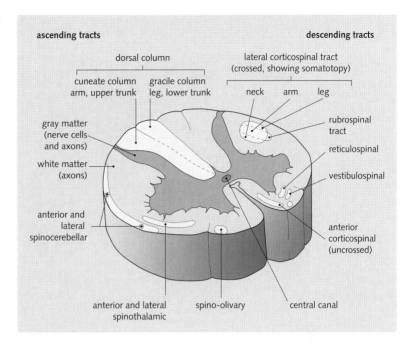

This pathway:
- Segregates information into modality-specific pathways for touch, hair movement, pressure, and joint rotation.
- Contains feedback mechanisms to gate the amount of incoming information to the cortex.

These functions are carried out in the areas where the pathway is interrupted by synapses, to allow for reorganization, segregation, and suppression. Fig. 3.4 shows the dorsal column system as a three-neuron pathway. The first neurons in the pathway synapse in the dorsal column nuclei (gracile and cuneate).
- Sensory input from the leg and lower trunk travels to the gracile nucleus.
- Sensory input from the arm, upper trunk, and neck to the cuneate nucleus.
- Sensory input from the face goes via the trigeminal nerve (cranial nerve V) to the trigeminal nucleus.

The next synapse is in the contralateral ventroposterolateral nucleus of the thalamus (or VPL) or the contralateral ventroposteromedial nucleus (VPM) for trigeminal inputs. The inputs reach here via the medial lemniscus.

The homuncular organization which began in the dorsal columns and trigeminal nuclei is amplified

here and reaches its climax in the cortex. The neurons from the VPL and VPM nuclei project to the cortex via the thalamocortical radiations.

Spinothalamic tract and pain signals

In addition to pain, the spinothalamic tract also carries crude touch and thermal information. Pain information is also carried in the spinoreticular and spinomesencephalic tracts.

Noxious and thermal information is carried into the dorsal horn by fast myelinated Aδ fibers (conveying sharp, stabbing pain) and slower unmyelinated C fibers (conveying dull, nagging pain as well as thermal information).

Aδ fibers terminate in laminae I and V. The axons from these cells cross over to the opposite side of the cord (decussate) and ascend in the anterolateral white matter, forming the spinothalamic tract.

C fibers influence the firing of the spinothalamic dorsal horn cells via interneurons, because they terminate in a different layer of the cord—lamina II. This provides further synaptic steps in the pain pathway, which may comprise targets for modulation of pain signal transmission by higher centers.

Fig. 3.5 shows that the spinothalamic fibers join the medial lemniscus in the medulla and project to the thalamus. The thalamic termination of the tract is in the ventroposterior nuclei and also in the

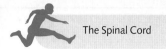

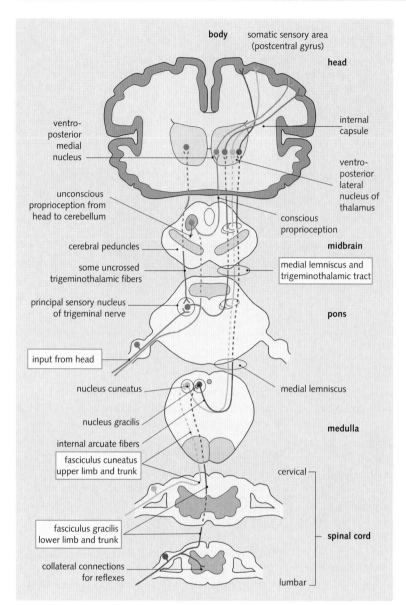

Fig. 3.4 The dorsal column pathway for touch and proprioception. The system is a three-neuron pathway with a synapse in the medulla, thalamus, and cortex. Note the decussation in the medulla.

intralaminar nuclei, from which there is a relay to the cortex.

As with fine touch, nociceptive afferent nerves from the face are carried in the trigeminal (V) nerve to the spinal trigeminal nucleus (which takes over the function of dorsal horn laminae I and II). The ascending fibers from the spinal nucleus of V cross over to the other side of the medulla and pass up to the thalamus to join the nociceptive spinothalamic inputs from the rest of the body.

Noxious input also projects to a variety of brainstem structures, some of which are implicated in generating sensations of agonizing pain (spinomesencephalic) and others being involved in arousal mechanisms (spinoreticular).

Spinocerebellar tract

The spinocerebellar tract (Fig. 3.6) deals with proprioceptive information and can be divided into two parts:

- The dorsal spinocerebellar tract is formed by the axons of cell bodies that lie in a column at the base of the dorsal horn (Clarke's column) running from T1 to L2. These cells receive information from

Fig. 3.5 The spinothalamic tract. Note the decussation at the same spinal level as the afferent fibers enter the cord.

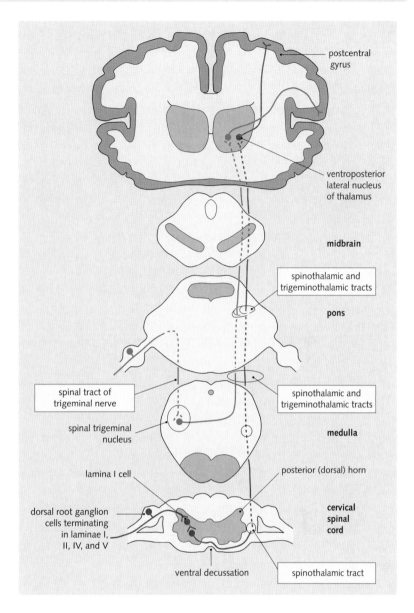

cerebellum via the superior cerebellar peduncle where most of the axons cross over again. This tract sends information primarily about inhibitory interneuron activity.

Descending pathways
The corticospinal tract

The corticospinal (sometimes called the pyramidal) tract is the major controller of skeletal muscle activity. It has two branches:

- The decussating lateral tract controls the precision movements of the limbs (innervating lateral motor neuron pools).

muscle spindles and tendon organs. Below L2, the fibers ascend in the dorsal columns before they synapse with the cells in Clarke's column. This tract conveys information about body movement, from the trunk and lower limb, to the cerebellum via the inferior cerebellar penduncle. The same kind of information from the upper limb is transferred via the external cuneate nucleus located laterally in the medulla.

- The ventral spinocerebellar tract receives its input from cell bodies in lamina VII (the spinal interneuron layer). Most of the axons cross to the other side of their segment, then up to the

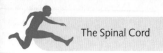

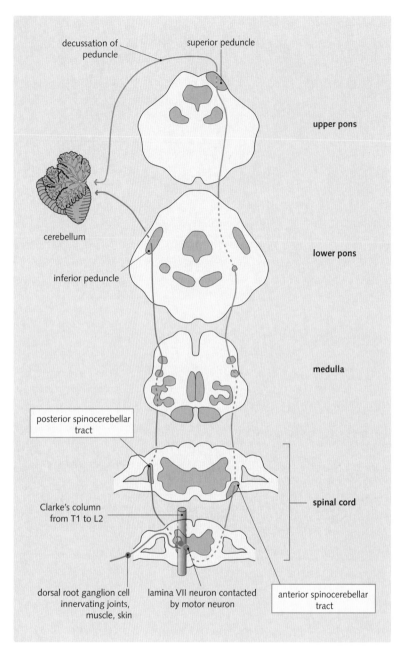

Fig. 3.6 The anterior and lateral spinocerebellar tracts.

- The uncrossed anterior tract controls the less precise movements of the trunk (innervating medial motor neuron pools).

The fibers that influence motor neurons innervating muscles in the head (e.g., extraocular muscles, tongue muscles, and facial muscles) run in the corticobulbar tracts to the appropriate cranial nerve nuclei. The somatotopic arrangement of the descending motor fibers from the cortex includes the head in the cerebral peduncles, but not at the level of decussation in the medulla (Fig. 3.7).

The motor fibers carry signals for highly skilled voluntary movements. To achieve this:
- The tract needs to be highly somatotopic.
- The fibers must have few collaterals so that excitation from one fiber is communicated to the minimum number of spinal motor neurons (this

Fig. 3.7 The corticospinal and corticobulbar tracts. Note the decussation in the spinal cord.

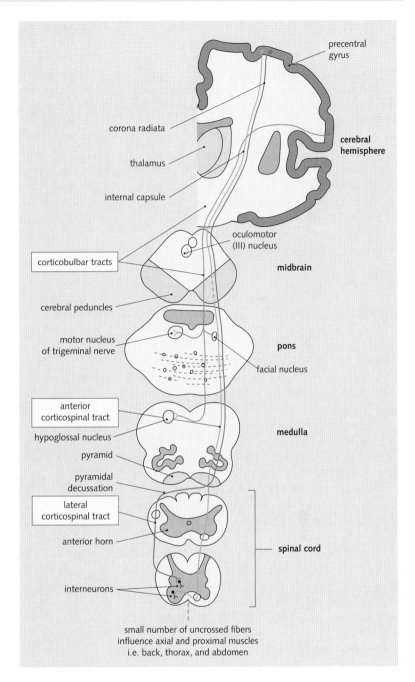

precentral gyrus

corona radiata

cerebral hemisphere

thalamus

internal capsule

oculomotor (III) nucleus

corticobulbar tracts

midbrain

cerebral peduncles

motor nucleus of trigeminal nerve

pons

facial nucleus

anterior corticospinal tract

hypoglossal nucleus

medulla

pyramid

pyramidal decussation

lateral corticospinal tract

anterior horn

spinal cord

interneurons

small number of uncrossed fibers influence axial and proximal muscles i.e. back, thorax, and abdomen

allows a great deal of control over the execution of movement).

As well as motor axons, there are fibers that regulate spinal reflexes in the tract and feedback to the dorsal horn sensory circuits from the sensory cortex.

Upper and lower motor neuron lesions

Damage to the motor cortex leads to an absence of volitional movement, but experimental evidence from cutting just the pyramidal tract in the medulla of monkeys results in very little motor deficit.

In humans, damage to the motor cortex and premotor areas after a cerebrovascular accident (or stroke) in the middle cerebral artery territory leads to a set of symptoms and signs affecting some of the contralateral muscles in the limbs and face. Because upper (i.e., cortical) motor neurons are involved, the effect is termed an "upper motor neuron lesion," although other cells are involved too.

Voluntary paresis (weakness) is caused by loss of corticospinal input. The symptoms and signs are:

- Spasticity or abnormal distribution in muscle tone which affects flexors more than extensors (this may be caused by disruption of extrapyramidal systems).
- Stronger deep reflexes (e.g., knee jerk).
- Loss of superficial reflexes (e.g., abdominal, cremasteric).
- Positive Babinski's sign—extensor plantar response to stroking the lateral part of the sole from heel to toe.

The effects of an upper motor neuron lesion are typically seen on the side of the body contralateral to the lesion. If there is localized damage to the motor cortex or pyramidal tract, all the input to an area will be affected due to homuncular and somatotopic organization.

Damage to the spinal motor neurons, either in the cord or along their pathway to the site of innervation of the muscle, produces a different set of symptoms and signs, referred to as a lower motor neuron lesion:

- Weakness caused by loss of nervous innervation.
- Atrophy as a result of disuse (this is a late sign).
- Fasciculation (squirming movements of the muscle) caused by increased sensitivity at receptor level to any acetylcholine that is released from intact terminals.
- Absent reflexes caused by loss of reflex output.

Other descending tracts

The other descending tracts are more involved in automatic or involuntary control of movement. They largely deal with the axial and proximal muscles which control posture.

The tectospinal tract controls head and neck posture. The tract begins with cells in the superior colliculus and their axons cross the midline in the midbrain, but only go as far as motor neurons in the cervical cord.

The vestibulospinal tract acts with the tectospinal to keep the head balanced on the shoulders as the body moves through space and to turn the head in response to sensory stimuli.

The reticulospinal tract (Fig. 3.8) controls posture and helps in the control of crude imprecise movements. The reticular formation is a term used to describe a diffuse network of cells in the brainstem which receives information from a large part of the central nervous system and is involved in the control of many of the body's automatic processes. There are two tracts of note:

- The pontine reticulospinal tract projects to motor neurons innervating axial muscles (in control of trunk posture).
- The medullary reticulospinal tract projects to motor neurons innervating distal muscles (in control of antigravity muscles).

The rubrospinal tract is thought to act as a parallel pathway to the corticospinal tract. Output from the

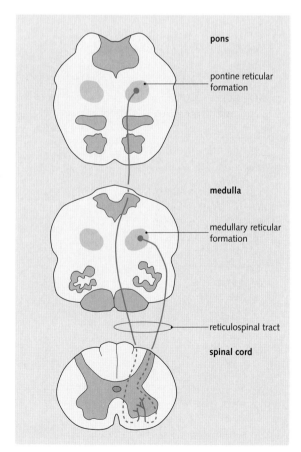

Fig. 3.8 The reticulospinal tract.

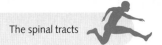

motor cortex travels both directly to the spinal cord and also via the red nucleus. Fibers from the red nucleus cross the midline in the pons and join the corticospinal tract.

Damage

Damage to the cord at different levels will produce different degrees of deficit in both motor and sensory function.

- Hemisection through the cord (Brown–Séquard syndrome) affects the ipsilateral spinothalamic, dorsal column, and corticospinal tracts. Symptoms and signs include no pain and temperature sensation below the lesion on the contralateral side, no fine touch or position sense below the lesion on the ipsilateral side, and weakness of the ipsilateral body below the lesion with the same distribution of upper motor neuron signs.
- Tabes dorsalis (tertiary syphilis) affects the dorsal columns bilaterally. Symptoms and signs include no perception of fine touch bilaterally and no proprioceptive feedback about movement bilaterally below the level of the lesion, which results in a stamping gait that produces mechanical damage to joints. Pain sensation is not affected.
- Syringomyelia (cavitation from the central canal into gray and white matter) initially affects the

After transection of the spinal cord, there may be an initial period where no reflexes can be elicited below the level of the lesion (when you would expect exaggerated reflexes). This coincides with a period of "spinal shock," which may persist for several weeks.

spinothalamic tract bilaterally and may extend to include motor neurons in the anterior horn and corticospinal tract. Symptoms and signs include bilateral loss of pain and temperature sensation below the lesion with variable degrees of lower motor neuron (anterior horn) signs. Fine touch perception is not affected.
- Complete section through the the whole cord (trauma, transverse myelitis) affects all tracts below the level of the lesion. Symptoms and signs include paralysis with upper motor below the level of the lesion. There is no sensation in any modality below the level of the lesion.
- Lesions to the VPL nucleus in the thalamus and somatosensory cortex show similar deficits to dorsal column lesions, but on the contralateral side of the body.

- Where can a lumbar puncture needle be inserted in the adult with the smallest risk of damage to the spinal cord?
- What are the differences between the dorsal and ventral columns?
- What are Rexed's laminae?
- Explain the three-neuron relay in the dorsal column pathway.
- What information is transferred in the spinocerebellar tracts?
- Describe the corticospinal tract and its two branches.
- How would you distinguish an upper motor neuron lesion from a lower motor neuron lesion?

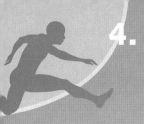

4. Somatosensation and the Perception of Pain

In this chapter, you will learn about:
- Somatosensation and the primary sensory cortex.
- Nociception and the perception of pain.
- Common analgesics and local anesthetics.

Somatosensation and the sensory cortex

Sensation

Sensation is a remarkably important part of life. Patients who have lost sensation in some way end up unable to perform simple tasks such as undoing buttons and manipulating coins. In severe forms of sensory disturbance (such as the neuropathy that occurs with diabetes), patients may sustain severe injuries—particularly to the feet in diabetics—partly because they cannot feel pain.

There are four sensory modalities—touch, thermal sensation, pain, and proprioception. In this chapter we shall not review proprioception, which is covered in Chapter 5.

There are individual receptors for submodalities within these groups. For example, the body can differentiate between light touch and pressure, between hot and cold, and between mechanical and thermal pain.

In humans, no matter how a receptor is activated (electrically or physiologically), the subjective sensation reported is always that of its modality. This has proven particularly useful for physiologists studying these processes! They have shown that there are modality-specific channels that convey information of one modality from the skin to the sensory receiving area.

Receptors

Receptors are formed by the peripheral terminations of the peripheral processes of dorsal root ganglion cells.

Receptors in the skin may be free nerve endings, or associated with different connective-tissue structures (e.g., Pacinian corpuscles).

Receptors can be divided into slowly adapting and rapidly adapting types. These two categories work in harmony to send different information about the same stimulus. The difference in signaling depends either on the linkage of the receptor to its incident energy or on a property called adaptation (i.e., a decline in receptor responsiveness even though the stimulus is still present and its intensity unchanged). As a general rule, slowly adapting receptors signal the magnitude or location of a stimulus, whereas rapidly adapting receptors signal its rate of change and duration.

The receptor membrane depolarizes in response to its modality stimulus, causing a generator potential. If sufficient, this causes the peripheral process (functional axon) to depolarize to its threshold level and produce an action potential. Because the fiber recovers after its refractory period, a long-lasting generator potential will cause the peripheral process to fire a train of impulses whose frequency will be proportional to the magnitude of the generator potential. To accommodate the wide range of sensory experience, different unimodal receptors have different thresholds, and the generator potential has a logarithmic relationship between stimulus intensity, frequency of firing, and ultimately perceived sensation.

Fig. 4.1 shows different fiber types for different modalities and their conduction speeds and fiber diameters.

The fibers leading centrally from these receptors enter the spinal cord via the dorsal roots, with the fibers signaling modalities of touch traveling in the dorsal column pathway, and the fibers signaling thermal and pain information traveling in the spinothalamic tract along with information about crude (poorly localized) touch. The dorsal column pathway and spinothalamic tract are discussed in detail in Chapter 3.

The site of the somatosensory cortex and its organization are shown in Fig. 4.2. The homunculus is distorted because more of the cortex is used to process information from certain body areas than others. Areas of greatest receptor density (i.e., other than free nerve endings) have the largest representation in the somatosensory cortex.

The somatosensory cortex has a homunculus for each modality (i.e., there is a map for touch, another

Fig. 4.1 Sensory afferent fibers.

Sensory afferent fibers				
Class	Modality	Axonal diameter (μm)	Conduction speed (m/s)	Pattern of termination in Rexed's laminae
myelinated				
Aα	proprioceptors from muscles, tendons	20	120	III, IV, V
Aβ	mechanoreceptors from skin	10	60	III, IV, V
Aδ	nociceptor, cold thermoreceptor	2.5	15	I, II, V
unmyelinated				
C	nociceptor, heat thermoreceptor	<1	<1	I, II

for pressure, etc., all lying next to each other). Within each homunculus, there is a columnar organization from the cortical surface to the underlying subcortical white matter. Within each column, the cells have similar receptive fields and modality specificity. The layers in the column send and receive fibers from different areas of the cortex and thalamus. This is shown in Fig. 4.3.

Nociception

Nociception is the sensory process that detects tissue damage. Pain is the perception of irritating, sore, stinging, throbbing, or painful sensations arising from the body. The way the body perceives pain not only depends on nociceptor input, but also on other pathways giving information about, for example, emotional components. Thus, pain is said to be an "experience" rather than a simple sensation.

Although nociceptors do not show adaptation (i.e., they fire continuously to tissue damage), pain sensation may come and go and pain may be felt in the absence of nociceptor discharge. Pain receptors rely on chemical mediators around the nerve ending which indicate tissue damage. Pain is also somehow related to itch. Itch is also mediated by Aδ and C fibers; people born without a sense of pain show no sense of itch, but interestingly, itch is unaltered by opiate (pain-relieving) drugs.

Hyperalgesia is the phenomenon of increased sensitivity of damaged areas to painful stimuli:

- Primary hyperalgesia occurs within the damaged area.
- Secondary hyperalgesia occurs in undamaged tissues surrounding this area.

After tissue damage occurs, blood vessels become leaky and the damaged tissue cells release a variety of chemicals that give a local response—inflammation (e.g., histamine, which directly excites nociceptors, and prostaglandin, which sensitizes nociceptors).

Nociceptor afferent fibers release not only the excitatory transmitter glutamate (as do all sensory afferent nerves), but also the cotransmitter substance-P. This causes a very long-lasting excitatory postsynaptic potential and helps sustain the effect of noxious stimuli.

Processing of nociceptive afferent signals begins in the circuits in the dorsal horn and a certain amount of descending control is exercised over the firing of spinothalamic cells in lamina I of the dorsal horn. Pain information is then transmitted to the thalamus and somatosensory cortex in the spinothalamic tract (see Chapter 3). Whether the cortex is the ultimate site of pain perception is a matter for debate. Certainly, subjects who are awake during neurosurgery do not report pain sensations when electrodes are passed through areas of the cortex. When those areas are stimulated, subjects may report tingling or thermal sensation, but not pain. It

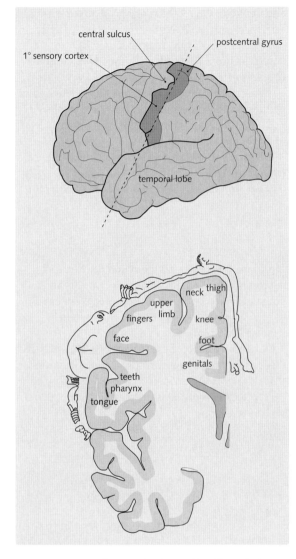

Fig. 4.2 Homuncular organization and location of primary sensory cortex (S1).

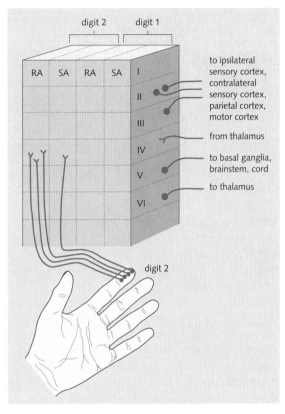

Fig. 4.3 Columnar organization of primary sensory cortex (RA, rapidly adapting; SA, slowly adapting).

is likely then that the conscious sensation of pain has a functionally significant subcortical component.

Referred pain

Pain from internal organs (viscera) is often felt as pain in a more superficial region of the body surface rather than in the visceral organ. Nociceptor sensory fibers from viscera and those from cutaneous structures converge on the same dorsal horn neurons that contribute to the spinothalamic tract. The central nervous system can make no distinction between superficial pain (somatic) and deep pain (visceral) and consequently interprets all pain as originating from the superficial (somatic) body part. For example:

- Pain of myocardial infarction is classically perceived as a radiating pain down the left arm and up the root of the neck into the jaw.
- Inflammation affecting the diaphragm is felt in the suprascapular (shoulder) region (phrenic nerve roots C3–C5).

Regulation of pain
Peripheral regulation

Pain can be regulated by sensory input—it can be reduced by activity in low-threshold (large fiber) mechanoreceptors as their afferent fibers inhibit spinothalamic cell discharge, the phenomenon of "rubbing it makes it better."

Transcutaneous electrical nerve stimulation (TENS) can be used to activate large-diameter fibers to decrease the sensation of pain. This is particularly useful in chronic pain states (e.g., lower back pain) and increasingly is being used as noninvasive pain relief for women in labor.

Central regulation

Pain can sometimes be suppressed by "willing it to go away." A possible reason for this is that there are regions in the central nervous system that have been implicated in pain suppression (Fig. 4.4).

Electrical stimulation of the periaqueductal gray matter in the midbrain causes profound analgesia. This area receives information from higher structures processing emotional states and projects to the midline reticular and raphe nuclei, which in turn project to the dorsal horn. Two other parts of the reticular formation—the nucleus reticularis paragigantocellularis and the locus coeruleus—are also implicated in modulating nociceptive neuronal activity in the dorsal horns.

Opiates are thought to produce their antinociceptive action by activating these central regulating structures.

Some of these regions contain endogenous opioid peptides, although pain modulation also involves 5-hydroxytryptamine (5-HT) from the raphe nuclei and noradrenaline from the locus coeruleus.

There are three classes of endogenous peptides (shown in Fig. 4.5).

There are three major classes of opioid receptor:
- μ (mu)
- δ (delta)
- κ (kappa)

Morphine is a potent μ-agonist and naloxone an antagonist. Endogenous enkephalins are active at both μ and δ receptors. Both receptor types are found in the periaqueductal gray matter and in laminae I and II of the dorsal horn.

Note that each of these receptors is found throughout the central nervous system, suggesting that they are involved in processes other than pain perception. This explains the other effects of opiates, such as euphoria and hallucinations.

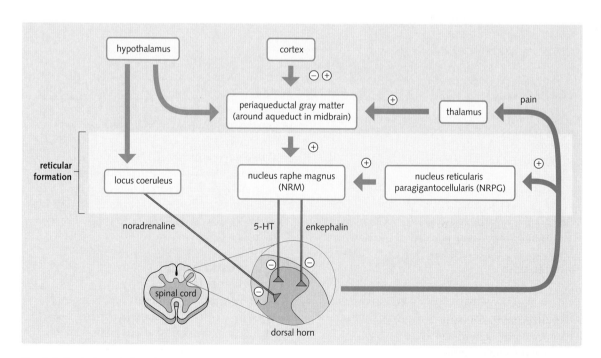

Fig. 4.4 Central regulation of pain.

Fig. 4.5 Opioid peptides.

Opioid peptides			
Parent peptide	Opioid peptide	Amino and sequence	Location
proenkephalin	enkephalins	Leu^5, Met^5, and longer sequences	spinal cord, brainstem
prodynorphin	dynorphins	all conain Leu^5 within longer sequences	spinal cord, brainstem
pro-opiomelanocortin	β-endorphin	Met^5 in 31 amino acid sequence	hypothalamus

Analgesia

Analgesia is relief from the psychological state of pain, whereas antinociception is simply the blockage of nociceptive inputs. The main analgesics in clinical use are:

- Opioid analgesics acting on the endogenous system of pain control.
- Nonsteroidal anti-inflammatory drugs, which reduce the production of inflammatory mediators that sensitize nociceptors to bradykinin and 5-HT.
- Simple analgesics (e.g., paracetamol).
- Local anaesthetics, which block action potential conduction along axons.
- Miscellaneous drugs (e.g., sumatriptan, a 5-HT$_{1D}$ agonist) in migraine; carbamazepine (antiepileptic) in trigeminal neuralgia; tricyclic antidepressants (amitryptyline) in some types of chronic pain.

Opioids

Opioid drugs bind to the receptors of the endogenous opioid transmitters. There are two classes of opioids:

- Opiates, which include morphine and analogs that are structurally similar to morphine and usually synthesized from it (e.g., diamorphine, codeine).
- Synthetic derivatives structurally unrelated to morphine (e.g., pethidine, fentanyl).

Opioids block pain information from being transmitted up the spinothalamic tract (antinociceptive action) but they also act in the brain to reduce the unpleasantness of the pain state (analgesic action).

- The weaker opioids (such as codeine) are widely used in over-the-counter pain preparations, and often in conjunction with a simple analgesic in prescription medications (e.g., co-codamol is codeine and paracetamol).
- Stronger opioids (such as morphine and pethidine) are used in postoperative pain and sometimes in severe chronic pain (such as cancer pain).
- Either fentanyl or morphine is commonly used as part of general anesthesia.

The main effect of opioids is on the μ receptor, causing:

- Analgesia and antinociception.
- Euphoria and drowsiness—depending on the circumstances of administration.
- Respiratory depression—reducing the sensitivity of the brainstem to $PaCO_2$.
- Miosis—pupillary constriction caused by stimulation of the parasympathetic component of cranial nerve III.
- Nausea—stimulation of the chemoreceptor trigger zone in the brainstem which sends signals to the vomiting center.
- Constipation—increased tone and reduced motility of gastrointestinal tract.

There are problems with repeated administration of opioids:

- Tolerance—a gradual reduction in effect over repeated administration of the same amount of drug. Doses of morphine therefore need to be increased over time to produce the same degree of

pain relief, but this causes a greater degree of constipation.
- Dependence—this can be physical (where a withdrawal syndrome of physical symptoms and signs like influenza occurs when the drug is not administered) or psychological (where compulsive drug-seeking behavior develops). Often, it is a combination of both.

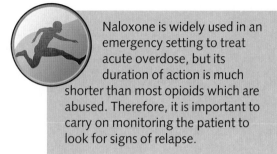

Naloxone is widely used in an emergency setting to treat acute overdose, but its duration of action is much shorter than most opioids which are abused. Therefore, it is important to carry on monitoring the patient to look for signs of relapse.

The opiate class of opioids (morphine, diamorphine, codeine) also inhibit histamine release from mast cells and are cough suppressants, but these effects are not mediated by opioid receptors. This is exploited by codeine-based cough medications.

The most common drug of abuse in this class is diamorphine (otherwise known as heroin), but it should be remembered that many patients will be taking opioids which are legitimately prescribed and will develop these side effects and may be at risk from overdose.

The main danger of opioid abuse is from overdose, which presents with:
- Coma.
- Respiratory depression.
- Pinpoint pupils (there is no tolerance to pupillary constriction even in the hardened addict).

Treatment is with intravenous μ-antagonists, such as naloxone (rapidly acting and short duration of action) or naltrexone (longer to act but longer duration of action). Note that antagonists may stimulate an acute withdrawal state and supportive therapy alone (e.g., ventilation) may be appropriate in some cases of opioid overdose.

The main opioids are shown in Fig. 4.6 with their different pharmacological properties and clinical uses.

Nonsteroidal anti-inflammatory drugs

Nonsteroidal anti-inflammatory drugs relieve pain by reducing the sensitization of nociceptors that occurs in inflammation. NSAIDs are also anti-inflammatory and antipyretic (decrease fever). They inhibit:
- Cyclooxygenase (which metabolizes arachidonic acid to prostaglandins).
- Leukotrienes (which have roles in continuing the process of inflammation).

The prostaglandins, PGE_1 and PGE_2, lower the threshold of polymodal nociceptors to stimulation by the inflammatory mediators bradykinin and 5-HT.

The production of prostaglandins in these normal circumstances is by a subtype of cyclooxygenase, cyclooxygenase-1. The other type, cyclooxygenase-2 (COX-2), is inducible and metabolizes arachidonic acid in inflammatory cells. Side effects of these drugs can result from interference with the physiological role of prostaglandins in the regulation of blood flow. For example, interfering with blood flow in the gastric mucosa reduces HCO_3^- production. Gastric acid can then attack the mucosal surface causing ulceration and potentially fatal bleeding.

This has led to the introduction of selective COX-2 inhibitors which are marketed as being less damaging to the gastric mucosa.

Fig. 4.7 shows the main NSAIDs in clinical use with their effects and side effects. Fig. 4.8 shows the site of action of NSAIDs.

Generally, NSAIDs are considered to be very safe drugs and are widely available. However, aspirin use has been linked to Reye's syndrome in children (causing liver damage and encephalopathy after a viral illness). Chronic NSAID use may also cause an interstitial nephritis, with lasting kidney damage in some patients.

5. Motor Control

In this chapter, you will learn about:
- The control of movement.
- Proprioception.
- Motor units and the control of muscle.
- The motor cortex.
- The basal ganglia.
- The cerebellum.

Movement control

Types of movement
There are three basic types of movement:
- Reflex responses (e.g., the gag reflex)—stereotyped, involuntary responses graded to the intensity of the eliciting stimulus.
- Rhythmic motor patterns (e.g., walking)—sequences of stereotyped repetitive responses that are largely automatic, but that require voluntary control to start and stop.
- Voluntary movements—these are goal-directed, usually learned, and improved with practice.

Movements may also be categorized according to their speed: slow or ramp movements are controlled by sensory feedback, very fast or ballistic movements are not.

Muscle contraction is used to produce stabilization of the body (to provide the correct posture against gravity), as well as to produce movement.
- If the external force is smaller than that produced by the muscle, then movement occurs and an isotonic contraction is produced.
- When the external force is greater than that produced by the muscles an isometric contraction is produced.
- If the external force is greater than the muscle contraction, then muscle lengthening occurs as is the case in walking down a flight of stairs.

The importance of sensation
Sensory information can be used in a feedback or feedforward control system.
- In feedback control, the nervous system generates a movement and sensory information is used to

obtain an error signal, which is the difference between the desired position and the current position. It is the sense of proprioception, which provides information about the position of the body (joints and muscles) and the movements of muscle groups. These sensations are transferred to the brain in both the dorsal column tract and the spinocerebellar tract. Patients who have lost their sense of proprioception due to a large-fiber sensory neuropathy do not know where their limbs are in space unless they can see them.
- In feedforward control, sensory information is used to derive advance information and direct the movement toward a predicted position (e.g., picking up a drink).

Motor programs and voluntary movement
Definitions
A "motor program" is a sequence of nerve impulses that, when sent to a group of muscles, will execute a movement. The same motor program can be scaled and timed differently and sent to different muscle groups—for example, it is possible to hold a pen and write with either hand (with different levels of success!).

A "motor strategy" is a set of motor programs that have been selected and sequenced to achieve a recognized goal. An example of this may be playing a tennis shot. A motor program is needed for the arm holding the racket, the legs to give the correct footwork, and to the trunk muscles to give the correct swing.

Development of motor programs
Motor programs are time-saving for the motor system because they enable fast accurate movement.

The following stages in the process of learning motor programs show how proprioceptive feedback is used to adjust the motor output until the precise motor commands are developed. As a motor task is learned, the pattern of muscle activity changes.
- Initially, discontinuous movement occurs where the muscles working to achieve the task (agonists) move the limb nearer and nearer toward a target, judging the end-point with feedback. This yields a

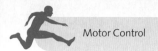

relatively slow movement, which may not be terribly smooth.

- Faster, continuous movement then develops, with a single agonist burst stopped by an antagonist, then smaller adjustments guided by feedback made with agonist muscles. This is a smoother movement, which comes closer to the target in a shorter time.
- Eventually, the movement becomes ballistic, with a single agonist burst to move the limb toward the target and a single antagonist burst to stop the limb moving so that it comes to rest at the target.

Hierarchy of movement control

There are three levels of motor control arranged hierarchically and in parallel. The lowest level is at the spinal cord. The interneurons in the cord play a major role in sequential operations of muscles that can produce complex movements under sensory control.

The intermediate level is at the brainstem containing medial, lateral, and aminergic systems. These project to and regulate segmental networks of the spinal cord and are responsible for the integration of visual, vestibular, and somatosensory inputs in the control of posture. In addition, some brainstem nuclei control eye and head movements.

The highest level is in the cortical control of voluntary movement.

- Processes that generate the desire to move in response to recognized demands can be localized to the frontal lobes and limbic system.
- Processes generating strategies to achieve motor aims, by selecting motor programs, can be localized to the combination of the premotor and supplementary motor areas. Each area projects to the primary motor cortex and then to the spinal motor neurons via the corticospinal tract. There is also an indirect pathway via the brainstem, which is arranged somatotopically both for input and output. The basal ganglia also have a role in motor planning in the scaling and initiation of motor programs.
- Processes that guide movement are carried out by the primary motor cortex and descending motor tracts. The pyramidal tract governs highly skilled movement involving few muscles. The cerebellum improves the accuracy of movements by comparing descending motor commands (intended movement) with information about resulting motor activity (actual movement), and

also helps to maintain body position through postural muscles.

- The process of execution of movement is carried out by spinal neurons that innervate skeletal muscle.

Motor units and the recruitment of muscle fibers

Motor units

A motor unit consists of a motor neuron and all the muscle fibers that it innervates. One motor neuron may innervate many muscle fibers but a single muscle fiber receives input from only one motor neuron (Fig. 5.1).

The innervation ratio of a motor unit is the number of muscle fibers innervated by a single motor neuron.

- A high innervation ratio means that one motor neuron controls many fibers—such a motor unit produces coarse strong movements (e.g., the motor units in gastrocnemius have a ratio of 1:2000).
- A low innervation ratio means that only a few fibers are controlled by a single motor neuron— such a motor unit produces fine, well-controlled movement (e.g., the motor units in the extraocular muscles have a ratio of 1:10).

Motor units differ in their functional properties owing to variation in types of motor neurons and variations in the types of muscle fibers innervated.

There are essentially two types of motor neurons—large α-motor neurons that innervate the skeletal muscle fibers directly, and smaller γ-motor neurons that innervate the intrafusal fibers of muscle spindles (see section on reflexes below).

Recruitment

Two functional types of motor units can be distinguished by their histochemical features:

- Fast twitch (pale) muscle fibers, involved in quick, phasic movements such as running and walking. This class can be further divided into fast fatigable and fast fatigue-resistant categories.
- Slow tonic (dark-red) muscle fibers, involved in slow sustained contractions, such as those involved in the maintenance of posture.

Muscles typically have a variable number of different types of motor units, as seen by staining techniques

Properties of motor neurons and function, histology, and biochemistry of muscle fibers			
Motor unit	Properties of motor neuron	Functional properties of muscle fibers	Histology and biochemistry of muscle fibers
slow fatigue-resistant	constant low-frequency firing rate with steady-sate depolarization; smaller cell body, smaller diameter axon with slower conduction velocity	longer contraction and relaxation times, lower force (10% of fast fatiguable), very resistant to fatigue	many mitochondria, high levels of oxidative enzymes (succinic dehydrogenase), high levels of myoglobin
fast fatigue-resistant	intermediate firing rate response to steady-state depolarization; intermediate cell body size, axon diameter, and conduction speed	slightly slower than fast fatiguable contraction and relaxation times, twice force of slow units, very resistant to fatigue	many mitochondria, high levels of glycolytic and oxidative enzymes, high levels of myosin ATPase
fast fatigable	progressive drop in firing rate with steady-state depolarization; large cell body, large-diameter axon with high conduction velocity	fast contraction and relaxation times, high force during tetanus, fatigue after repeated stimulation	few mitochondria, high levels of glycolytic enzymes (phosphorylase), high levels of myosin ATPase

Fig. 5.1 Properties of motor units—the firing characteristics of their motor neurons and properties of the muscle fibers.

that visualize enzymes (e.g., myosin ATPase). For example, postural muscles have many slow, dark-red fibers, whereas extraocular muscles have mainly fast, pale fibers.

Recruitment describes the order in which types of motor units are activated when making any movement, whether it is reflex or voluntary. Slow units are activated first, then fast fatigue-resistant units, and finally fast fatigable units.

This allows the motor system to grade the amount of force used in a movement. A small amount of excitatory input to a pool of different types of motor neurons in the anterior horn will only produce firing of the slow (lower threshold) motor neurons. Greater amounts of stimulation are required to activate the faster (higher threshold) and more powerful units.

Tetanic contraction

Tetanic contraction occurs when successive muscle contractions are so rapid that they fuse together resulting in a sustained contraction with maximal force. This phenomenon has only been seen *in vitro*.

Responses of motor units in damage and disease

Diseases affecting different parts of the motor unit disrupt its normal function, as shown by changes in

the pattern of motor unit arrangement, the size of muscle fibers, and electrical recordings from muscle fibers when active and at rest (electromyogram) (Fig. 5.2).

Repeated activation of muscle fibers causes depletion of intracellular ATP stores, meaning that the muscle produces less force. However, the fibers remain in a state of partial contraction for some time because relaxation is also an active process requiring ATP. This slow relaxation time has the effect of decreasing the force available to sustained contraction, but not that of single twitches (in early fatigue).

In myasthenia gravis, muscles (particularly those of the eyelid, neck, and shoulders) are particularly fatigable. This is caused by a defect in the neuromuscular junction where there are autoantibodies directed against the acetylcholine receptor. This fatigue can be temporarily overcome by the use of acetylcholinesterase inhibitors, which is the basis of the diagnostic Tensilon test.

Tetany occurs where hypocalcemia or alkalosis reduce the threshold for action potential generation and neurons fire spontaneously. Typically this produces muscle spasms in the hands such that the fingers and thumbs are adducted and the wrist flexed at the metacarpophalangeal joints. This should not be confused with tetanus, which is a disease caused by a

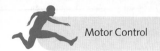

Clinical features and effects on motor units of diseases of the motor neuron cell body, peripheral axon, and muscle fiber

Part of motor unit affected	Typical clinical features	Example	Effect on muscle fibers	EMG changes
motor neuron cell body	weakness, atrophy affecting distal muscles more than proximal, fasciculation [lower motor neuron lesion signs although hyperreflexia is seen in amyotrophic lateral sclerosis (ALS)]	amyotrophic lateral sclerosis (motor neuron disease)	atrophy and disappearance of groups of muscle fibers, with other fibers innervated by new collaterals from remaining motor neurons; this produces "fiber clumping" where areas of muscle contain fibers of only one type (fiber type is determined by motor neuron type—response to disease results in collaterals of one motor neuron innervating many nearby fibers)	spontaneous activity at rest (fibrillation), discrete pattern of potentials during voluntary contraction as fewer motor units active, potentials are larger as motor units innervate more fibers than usual; no change in axon conduction velocity
motor neuron axon	chronically—weakness, atrophy distally, loss of tendon reflexes, sensory symptoms (loss, paraesthesia) as all types of peripheral nerve are affected	Guillain–Barré syndrome		fibrillation, discrete large potentials; demyelinating neuropathies (Guillain–Barré syndrome) result in reduced axon conduction velocity
muscle fiber	weakness initially affecting walking and lifting, proximal larger muscles involved more than distal ones	Duchenne's muscular dystrophy	no change in spread of type of motor unit; dead fibers and regenerating fibers are present; inflammatory cells and fat sometimes present	no spontaneous activity at rest, shorter smaller potentials as there are fewer remaining fibers in each motor unit; the overall pattern is still smooth as there is no reduction in the number of motor units firing

Fig. 5.2 Diseases affecting the motor neuron cell body, peripheral axon, and muscle fibers—clinical features.

toxin from a soil-dwelling bacterium. The symptoms of the latter disease include muscle contractions and "lockjaw"—it may be fatal if not swiftly treated.

Reflex action and muscle tone

Clinical relevance

Neurological examination of patients' limbs includes testing stretch reflexes. For example, tapping the patellar tendon and observing the result indicates whether the spinal cord segments L2 and L3 and their related spinal nerves are intact, and can also indicate if the spinal motor neurons are receiving an altered input from higher centers. When an upper motor neuron lesion is present, there is a loss of

descending inhibition of stretch reflexes and this results in hyperactive (or more brisk) tendon reflexes.

Passive movement of a limb provides the examiner with information about the tone of the muscles in the limb; the greater the tone, the more resistance to movement.

Definitions

"Reflex action" is an automatic motor response (simple or highly coordinated) that is elicited by a stimulus. The stretch reflex (such as that elicited by tapping the patellar tendon) is simple because the stretch detector (the muscle spindle) forms a monosynaptic connection with the output spinal motor neuron in the ventral horn. Other reflexes have neurons interposed between the sensory input and the motor output (interneurons) and can produce more complex responses. The magnitude of the reflex response can be influenced by higher centers.

"Muscle tone" is the term that refers to the resting tension in muscle. It is produced by tonic firing of spinal motor neurons whose firing frequency is determined by a combination of inputs from stretch receptors and from higher centers through corticospinal, vestibulospinal, and rubrospinal tracts.

> A stretch reflex can be "reinforced" by performing a Valsalva maneuver, pulling the hands outward against each other. This is useful in patients whose reflexes are hard to elicit.

In parkinsonism, muscles are said to be "rigid" and exhibit increased tone, but there is no change in the strength or speed of their reflexes.

A stroke may cause cell death in descending cortical motor neurons due to hemorrhage or ischemia. This leads to "spasticity" in skeletal muscles on the contralateral side, where tone is increased more in limb anti-gravity muscles, and this is known as a pyramidal distribution of weakness. In these patients, stretch reflexes elicit stronger responses, and this may produce stretch-induced rhythmic involuntary muscle contractions known as clonus. Reduced cortical input to the reflex circuit frees it from supraspinal inhibition and reflex activity is increased, and this is combined with increased muscle tone at rest.

Proprioceptors and reflexes
Muscle spindles

Spindles consist of thin skeletal muscle fibers enclosed in a connective tissue capsule (the fibers are called "intrafusal" muscle fibers; all the relatively large fibers outside the spindle are "extrafusal"). Only the distal ends of the intrafusal fibers contain contractile elements.

The distal portion of peripheral processes of dorsal root ganglion cells enter the capsule and innervate the noncontractile middle part of the intrafusal fibers. There are several varieties of these

sensory fibers and they are named according to their size and the arrangement of their nuclei:

- Nuclear chain intrafusal fibers have their nuclei distributed linearly in the central region of the fiber. The sensory endings of these fibers are sensitive to the absolute length of the muscle.
- Nuclear bag intrafusal fibers exhibit a central clump or aggregation of nuclei. The functional properties of these fibers can be described as dynamic (signaling the rate of change in the length of the muscle) or static (performing a function similar to the nuclear chain fibers, signaling muscle length) (Figs. 5.3 and 5.4).

Muscle spindle afferents can be described as either large myelinated fibers (group I) or small myelinated fibers (group II). Group Ia afferents that innervate muscle spindles have a slightly larger diameter than the Ib afferents that innervate Golgi tendon organs.

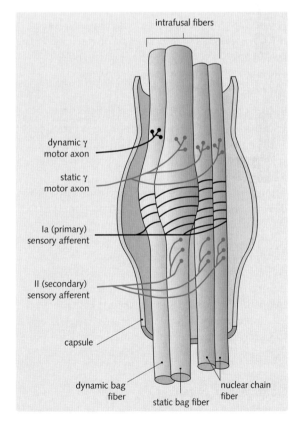

Fig. 5.3 Innervation and contents of a muscle spindle. Ia afferents are large, myelinated, fast fibers that are rapidly adapting. Type II afferents are small, myelinated, slower fibers that are slowly adapting.

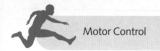

Properties of the two types of sensory ending from the muscle spindle			
Type	Contact	Response to linear stretch	Encoding
Ia (primary) ending	dynamic bag, static bag, nuclear chain		velocity of change of length, static length
II (secondary) ending	static bag, nuclear chain	stretch — release — time	static length

Fig. 5.4 Properties of the two types of sensory afferents found in the muscle spindle.

The contractile parts of the intrafusal fibers are innervated by γ-motor neurons which serve to alter the sensitivity of the intrafusal fibers to stretch and to the rate of change (velocity) in stretch. Dynamic γ-motor neurons innervate dynamic bag fibers and static γ-motor neurons innervate static bag and chain fibers. The γ-motor neuron is generally activated at the same time as the α-motor neuron (alpha-gamma coactivation) to ensure that both intra- and extrafusal fibers contract simultaneously.

Spindles and α-motor neuron firing

Increasing the activity of γ-motor neurons stimulates both contractile ends of the intrafusal fibers, thereby stretching the middle (nuclear region) of the fibers. The middle portion is enwrapped by stretch-receptor afferent fibers whose central processes form direct monosynaptic links with α-motor neurons in the spinal cord ventral horn. Therefore, α-motor neurons can be made to discharge by activation of γ-motor neurons and their related sensory fibers that complete the reflex loop.

Since α-motor neurons and γ-motor neurons are frequently activated together, the muscle spindle retains its sensitivity when the muscle is in use, and this provides very accurate feedback signals for error detection during voluntary movement.

Golgi tendon organs

Golgi tendon organs are found at the junction between muscle and tendon. They are composed of a network of collagen fibers inside a connective tissue capsule with a large, heavily myelinated type Ib sensory fiber winding around the collagen.

The firing rate of the Ib afferent fiber increases when the tendon organ is stretched, with greater outputs for active contraction rather than passive stretch of the muscle. These organs provide information mainly about active changes in tension in the muscle. Since their activation threshold is higher than that of muscle spindles, the signal may also be used to prevent injury to the muscle from excess tension.

Other receptors

There are various receptors present in joint capsules and ligaments that respond to length and changes in joint angle.

Examples of reflexes
Basic pattern

The stretch reflex is elicited when a muscle is suddenly lengthened and a reflex contraction is produced (e.g., tapping the patellar tendon causing a reflex contraction of the quadriceps muscle). Homonymous motor neurons (supplying the same muscle) and synergist motor neurons (supplying a muscle with the same action) receive an excitatory input via the activated spindle (Ia) afferent fibers. The spindle afferents also inhibit antagonistic muscles via Ia inhibitory interneurons in the spinal cord.

Golgi tendon organs form part of a reflex circuit termed the inverse myotatic reflex that inhibits homonymous and synergistic motor neurons. The pathways for these reflexes are shown in Fig. 5.5.

Blink reflex

The blink reflex protects the cornea from foreign bodies (Fig. 5.6).

Fig. 5.5 Muscle spindle and Golgi tendon organ reflexes. Muscle spindles detect the rate of change and absolute muscle length during movement. Golgi tendon organs provide information on tension, and are particularly useful in exploratory movements as they have the protective effect of decreasing muscle force when resistance is met. They are modulated by higher centers to allow their response properties to be modified.

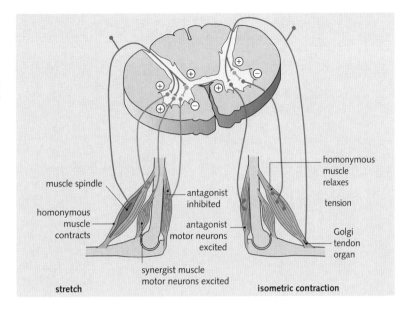

Fig. 5.6 Corneal (blink) reflex—protects the cornea from foreign bodies and other injuries.

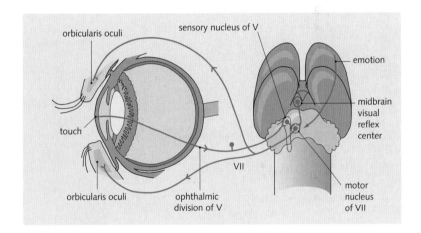

Gag reflex

The gag reflex protects the alimentary tract and upper airway from foreign bodies (Fig. 5.7).

Flexion withdrawal reflex

The flexion withdrawal reflex involves a more complicated circuit that protects limbs against potentially noxious stimuli detected by cutaneous pain receptors. The flexors of the affected limb contract and the extensors are relaxed. This withdraws the limb from the noxious stimulus.

At the same time, via excitatory contralaterally projecting interneurons, a crossed extensor reflex is elicited in the contralateral limb where the extensor muscles are contracted and flexors relaxed. This provides postural support during the withdrawal of the stimulated limb. In some instances, muscles in all four limbs can be involved in the reflex response as a result of multisegmental, ascending or descending connections formed by propriospinal (intersegmental) neurons whose axons course throught the fasciculus proprius that lies directly adjacent to the spinal cord gray matter.

Fig. 5.8 shows the polysynaptic pathways in the spinal cord with extensor and flexor action of stimulated and nonstimulated limbs.

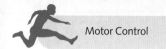

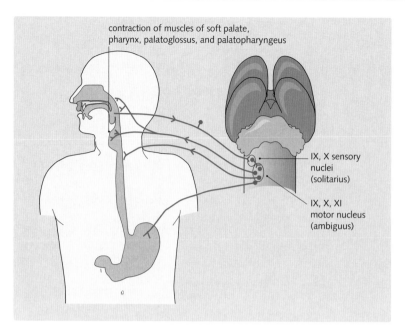

Fig. 5.7 Gag reflex showing a combination of skeletal muscle action (e.g., muscles of pharynx) and smooth muscle action (e.g., contraction of stomach).

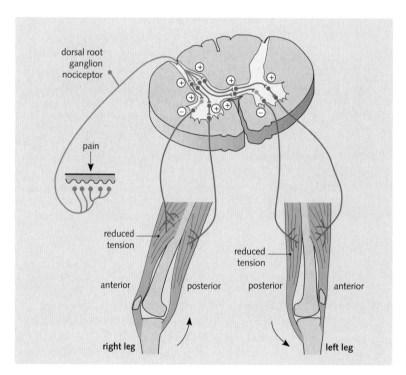

Fig. 5.8 The flexion withdrawal reflex showing withdrawal to pain on the left side, with a crossed extensor reflex in the right leg.

Plantar reflex

The plantar reflex is elicited when the plantar surface of the foot is stroked from heel to toe, causing reflex plantar flexion of the toes in normal individuals. However, in infants (whose corticospinal tract is not yet fully myelinated) and in patients with damage to the motor cortex or corticospinal tract (an upper motor neuron lesion), dorsiflexion of the toes is elicited. This is known as a positive Babinski sign.

The motor cortex

The motor cortex located in the frontal lobe (Fig. 5.9) is the area of the cortex that is involved in the planning and execution of motor commands.

The premotor area and supplementary motor area lie immediately anterior to the primary motor area which is localized to the precentral gyrus in the frontal lobe. It is believed that these two regions formulate the plan for movements because positron emission tomography scanning shows increased metabolism in the premotor area and supplementary motor area when the subject is asked to think about (but not execute) a movement. These areas are arranged according to a body (somatotopic) plan, the motor homunculus:

- The supplementary motor area projects to distal muscles and has a role in coordination of bimanual movements.
- The premotor area projects through reticulospinal and corticospinal tracts to proximal muscles.

Both areas receive input from motor regions that process different aspects of movement:
- The premotor area receives input from the cerebellum and basal ganglia via the thalamus, along with sensory inputs from the primary sensory and visual cortices.
- The supplementary motor area receives input from the basal ganglia through the thalamus, and also from the contralateral supplementary motor area.

Both areas also project to the primary motor area.

The primary motor area performs the final stage in cortical motor processing—execution. It projects to all contralateral body (spinal and cranial) motor neurons, but principally those controlling the digits, toes, and facial and vocalization muscles, and has a somatotopic organization. It receives input from other motor cortical regions and from the cerebellum. It also receives sensory input from the somatosensory cortex—the cortical area for muscle and joint sense abuts the primary motor cortex.

Movements are represented in multiple motor cortex homunculi in the various motor cortical areas and, although the term homunculus is an abstract concept, it suggests that there is a larger repertoire of movements for the hands, face, and vocal muscles than for the trunk.

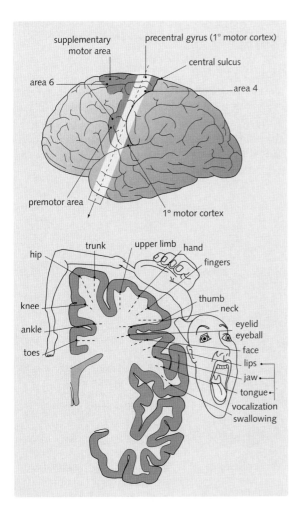

Fig. 5.9 Location and homuncular organization of the primary motor cortex.

In epileptic patients, disordered neuronal firing during a seizure can affect the motor cortex. This produces a wave of muscle activity, termed a "jacksonian march," that progressively and sequentially moves over the body as the disruption of function spreads across the motor cortex. This observation contributed to the original theories of homuncular (somatotopic) organization in the motor cortex.

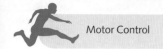

Basal ganglia and thalamus

Overview

The basal ganglia consist of five cell groups with extensive connections, which are involved in motor control and cognition. They are functionally inserted in several processing loops with the cortex and thalamus. Basal ganglia function is further understood by relating the signs of Parkinson's and Huntington's disease to the affected parts of the basal ganglia.

Anatomy

Fig. 1.4 (Chapter 1) shows the relationship between the putamen, caudate nucleus, and all the elements of the basal ganglia.

Fig. 5.10 shows the thalamus as a football-shaped collection of cell groups with the thalami on either side separated by the space of the third ventricle and joined by the interthalamic adhesion which essentially forms a bridge across the third ventricle.

The thalamus is organized around a Y-shaped collection of white matter called the "internal medullary lamina." This splits the thalamus into three sections—the anterior, lateral, and medial portions. Each portion is composed of numerous cell groups with particular inputs and functions. There are also cell groups within the internal medullary lamina called the intralaminar nuclei.

Connections and circuits of the basal ganglia and thalamus

Caudate and putamen

The caudate and putamen contain identical cell types and together they form the main input-receiving complex of the basal ganglia. These two structures are collectivley referred to as the neostriatum (which is often truncated to "striatum"). They receive somatotopic information from motor, sensory, association, and limbic areas of the cortex, and also from the intralaminar nuclei of the thalamus.

The corticostriate projection is topographically and functionally organized so that the putamen is primarily concerned with motor control and the caudate with eye movements and cognition. They project to the globus pallidus and the substantia nigra.

Globus pallidus

The globus pallidus is divided into internal (GP_i) and external (GP_e) segments located immediately lateral to the internal capsule and medial to the putamen. The internal segment is the major output cell group that projects to the ventrolateral and ventral anterior

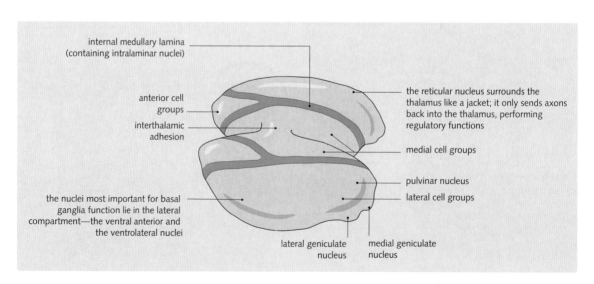

Fig. 5.10 The thalamus.

nuclei of the thalamus. The projection from the striatum to the GP_i, and from there to the thalamus, is known as the direct pathway.

Subthalamic nucleus

The subthalamic nucleus lies just inferior to the thalamus at its junction with the midbrain and receives a projection from, and projects back to, the external segment of the globus pallidus. It also has an excitatory output to the internal segment. The pathway linking the striatum to the GP_e, subthalamic nucleus, and the GP_i is known as the indirect pathway.

Substantia nigra

The substantia nigra lies in the midbrain and is divided into:

- A ventral pale part—pars reticulata, which projects to the ventrolateral and ventral anterior thalamic nuclei, and the superior colliculus.
- A dorsal pigmented part—pars compacta, which contains dopaminergic neurons and projects to the caudate and putamen as the nigrostriatal pathway.

The cellular interactions in the striatum are shown in Fig. 5.11.

Re-entrant processing loops

Figs. 5.12 and 5.13 show the direct and indirect processing loops that run through the basal ganglia. By working through each loop and examining the patterns of excitation and inhibition in each pathway, it can be seen that the direct loop excites cortical neurons via the thalamus while signals coursing through the indirect loop lead to inhibition of cortical neurons.

Functions of the basal ganglia

The basal ganglia select the motor programs that are appropriate for the execution of a particular task that might involve both cognitive and motor processing. Muscle activation required to perform the movement is controlled via the direct pathway while muscles that would interfere with performance of the desired movement are inhibited through activity in the indirect pathway. The basal ganglia circuits are most active in controlling learned, stereotypic movements.

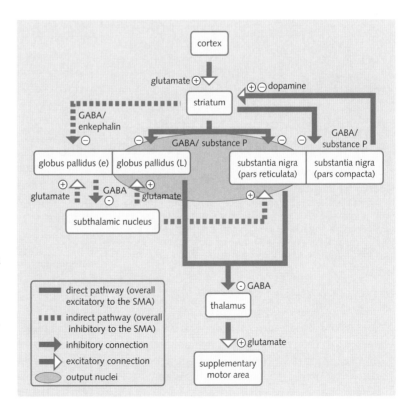

Fig. 5.11 Overview of the pathways through the basal ganglia with their neurotransmitters. Inhibitory signals from the output nuclei [GP_i and substantia nigra (pars reticulata)] cause decreased output to the supplementary motor area. The direct and indirect pathways are considered in subsequent simplified diagrams (Figs. 5.13 and 5.14, respectively) (GABA, γ-aminobutyric acid).

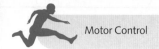

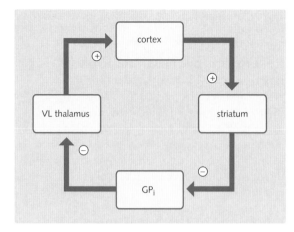

Fig. 5.12 The direct corticostriatal loop. When the striatum inhibits the internal globus pallidus (GP$_i$), it reduces the ability of the GP$_i$ to inhibit the thalamus. This effectively encourages the thalamus to fire, and to stimulate the cortex (supplementary motor area) (VL, ventrolateral).

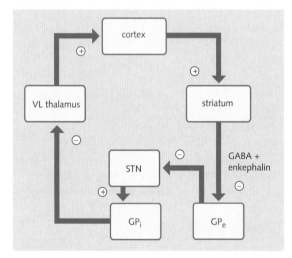

Fig. 5.13 The indirect loop. Striatal output inhibits the GP$_e$, reducing the inhibition of the subthalamic nucleus. The GP$_i$ is then excited by subthalamic neurons and in turn inhibits output from the VL thalamus. The cortex therefore receives less stimulation (GABA, γ-aminobutyric acid; VL, ventrolateral; GP$_e$, globus pallidus external segment; GP$_i$, globus pallidus internal segment).

The basal ganglia:
- Scale the output of the motor program so that appropriate movements are made. This is particularly important in motor programs involving fine movement (e.g., handwriting) and also where similar repetitive movements are needed (e.g., in locomotion).

- Project to the frontal eye fields via the thalamus, and have a role in the control of saccadic eye movements.
- Form connections with the prefrontal and other association cortices which may have a role in memory relating to body orientation.
- Are linked to the orbitofrontal cortex which suggests a role in modulating behavior.

Disorders involving basal ganglia function and their treatment
Parkinsonism
The signs resulting from decreased dopaminergic projections from the substantia nigra (pars compacta) to the striatum are collectively called "parkinsonism" and are due to an inability of the basal ganglia to process motor programs correctly. The signs include:
- Akinesia—poverty of movement, usually noticed first by lack of blinking and the appearance of a characteristic expressionless face (mask-like facial expression).
- Bradykinesia—when movement does occur it is abnormally slow.
- Tremor at rest—characteristically in the fingers and hands, it is called a "pill-rolling" tremor and has a frequency of 3–6 Hz.
- Rigidity—caused by increased tone in skeletal muscle that typically involves both flexors and extensors. When passive movement is attempted, the limbs move in a series of ratchety jerks. This is termed "cogwheel" rigidity.
- Micrographia—small handwriting results from inappropriate motor scaling.
- Shuffling gait—ambulation can be difficult to initiate but once started, its pace increases as the walking distance increases, termed a "festinating" gait.
- Abnormal postural reflexes producing a stooped, flexed total body posture.

Potential causes for the reduction in the dopaminergic projection to the caudate and putamen:
- Parkinson's disease is an idiopathic condition involving a progressive degeneration of dopaminergic neurons in the compact part of the substantia nigra which project to the striatum. Other cell groups are also affected—the ventral tegmental area (dopaminergic projection to ventral striatum), locus coeruleus (noradrenaline

projects diffusely throughout the central nervous system), and the raphe nuclei (5-hydroxytryptamine, which also project diffusely throughout the central nervous system).
- Postencephalitic parkinsonism.
- Neuroleptic medication taken for psychosis, which antagonizes the dopamine input to the striatum.
- Neurotoxin ingestion, infamously by drug addicts taking a synthetic morphine analog contaminated with MPTP (1-methyl-4-phenyl-1,2,3,6-tetrahydropyridine). This is metabolized by monoamine oxidase B to a compound MPP$^+$, which inhibits NADH dehydrogenase in dopaminergic terminals, reducing ATP production and promoting cell death.
- Exposure to and accumulation of certain herbicides.

The CNS attempts to compensate for the reduction in nigral dopaminergic cells by:
- Increasing the number of dopamine receptors in the striatum.
- Releasing more dopamine from the remaining neurons (shown as an increase in the levels of dopamine metabolites compared with dopamine levels).

The signs of parkinsonism occur when the compensatory mechanisms fail, but this occurs only after cell loss reaches approximately 80%. Drug treatment of parkinsonism (here restricted to the treatment of Parkinson's disease) aims to enhance the function of the remaining dopaminergic innervation to the striatum.

Antimuscarinics (e.g., benzhexol and benztropine)
The arrangement of striatal circuitry (Fig. 5.13) shows that nigral dopamine input inhibits striatal output cells while cholinergic striatal interneurons excite them. Thus, acetylcholine antagonists can be adminstered to compensate for reduced dopamine input. These agents can reduce tremor and rigidity but have little effect on bradykinesia. Side effects include drowsiness, confusion (which can exacerbate dementia in Parkinson's disease), and reduced parasympathetic function. Also, acetylcholine is not the only excitatory input to the striatum and this therapy is typically not effective for long.

Dopamine precursors
This approach bypasses the rate-limiting step of dopamine synthesis—tyrosine hydroxylase. L-Dopa, the drug of choice for most Parkinson's disease patients, is metabolized by dopa decarboxylase to dopamine. Dopamine itself cannot be given because it has many peripheral effects, and does not effectively cross the blood–brain barrier.

Side effects of L-dopa include:
- Nausea and vomiting caused by stimulation of D$_2$ receptors in the chemoreceptor trigger zone in the brainstem.
- Reduction in gastric emptying due to effects on gastric dopamine receptors.
- Dyskinesias—the striatum becomes overly sensitive to its dopamine input and overdose of L-dopa can occur producing involuntary movements, which are debilitating.
- Psychiatric effects (psychosis, depression, acute confusional state) due to nonselective alteration of all dopaminergic pathways that influence cortical function (e.g., ventral tegmental area to limbic system nuclei).

To increase the proportion of L-dopa reaching the central nervous system, other drugs need to be given to prevent L-dopa from being utilized by peripheral nervous structures such as sympathetic nerve terminals. Carbidopa and benserazide are inhibitors of dopa decarboxylase that act only in the periphery, as they do not cross the blood–brain barrier, and are an essential adjunct to L-dopa therapy.

In long-term treatment (>5 years):
- Deterioration is inevitable.
- Akinesia recurs.
- Drug tolerance develops, meaning equivalent doses give shorter periods of relief.
- The response to L-dopa becomes unpredictable.

Inhibitors of monoamine oxidase B
Inhibitors of monoamine oxidase B, such as selegiline, reduce the rate at which dopamine is degraded in nerve terminals and potentiate the effect of L-dopa. It is often reserved for severe disease when L-dopa is beginning to lose its efficacy.

Direct dopamine agonists
Direct dopamine agonists (e.g., bromocriptine) stimulate striatal receptors but do not mimic the normal conditions of dopamine release in the striatum. Side effects are similar to those of

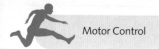

L-dopa—nausea and psychiatric disturbance. Again, they are reserved for severe disease.

Newer methods to treat Parkinson's disease include:

- Neurosurgery to ablate the hyperactive globus pallidus internal segment (pallidotomy).
- The placement of electrodes for deep brain stimulation in the globus pallidus internal segment and substantia nigra (pars reticulata) which depresses their function (via conduction block).
- Implantation of dopamine-rich brain tissue from aborted fetuses (this remains a controversial and, as yet, unproven therapy).

Huntington's disease

This autosomal dominant condition is caused by a defect on chromosome 4. It typically presents in midlife, but may show anticipation in subsequent generations. The symptoms are caused by selective cell death in the striatum of both acetylcholine- and GABA-containing neurons, particularly those that participate in the indirect pathway. Hyperkinesia develops with flailing dance-like or "choreic" movement. This is perhaps initially due to a loss of GABAergic striatal output cells projecting to the external globus pallidus. This releases the external pallidal segment neurons from inhibition and allows them to fire and produce inhibition of cells in the subthalamic nucleus. Consequently, there is a reduction of the excitatory output of the subthalamus to the internal pallidal segment resulting in the release of thalamocortical excitatory projections and the subsequent production of involuntary movements. Conceptually, this correlates very well with the fact that subthalamic lesions are known to produce contralateral involuntary movements (hemiballismus). Cognitive functions also deteriorate as striatal cell death continues, affecting the processing loops with the frontal lobes.

The cerebellum

Anatomy

The cerebellum is divided into four components—the flocculonodular lobe, the vermis, the intermediate zone, and the lateral cerebellar hemispheres.

The functional units include:

- The flocculonodular lobe (vestibulocerebellum) involved in the control of posture and eye movements.
- The vermis with the intermediate part of the hemisphere, or paravermis (together known as the spinocerebellum), involved in the control of both postural and distal muscles.
- The lateral part of the hemisphere (cerebrocerebellum) involved in coordination and planning of limb movements (in conjunction with the basal ganglia).

Fig. 5.14 shows the divisions of the cerebellum, including the central (deep) nuclei that integrate cerebellar cortical processing, forming an output that passes through the superior cerebellar peduncle.

Fig. 5.15 shows the folding of the cerebellar cortex into lobules and folia that give the cerebellum its furrowed appearance similar to the cerebral cortex.

Figs. 5.16 and 5.17 show the fundamental inputs to, and outputs from, the cerebellum.

The cerebellar cortex

The processing circuit in the cerebellar cortex, as shown in Fig. 5.18, can be divided into input axons, processing interneurons, and output neurons.

Mossy fibers from the spinocerebellar tract, the dorsal column nuclei, and the pontocerebellar fibers form the inputs, terminating on granule cells whose axons form the vast array of parallel fibers that synapse on Purkinje cell dendritic spines. Inputs from the inferior olivary nucleus in the brainstem (carrying information from the spino-olivary tract, brainstem, and cortex) enter the circuit as climbing fibers and make many synaptic contacts directly on Purkinje cell dendritic shafts. Climbing fibers from the spinal cord (via the inferior olive) also synapse directly with the Purkinje cells. Both parallel and climbing fibers also send inputs directly to the cerebellar nuclei prior to synapsing in the cerebellar cortex.

The interneurons in the circuit have different functions.

- Granule cells, which receive most of the input to the cortex from mossy fibers, send axons upward into the molecular layer nearest the cortical surface, branching in parallel and making many contacts with other cell types in the cortical circuit.
- Golgi cells, after receiving excitation from granule cells, inhibit them in a feedback loop.

Fig. 5.14 The posterior aspect of the cerebellum, showing the cerebellar nuclei.

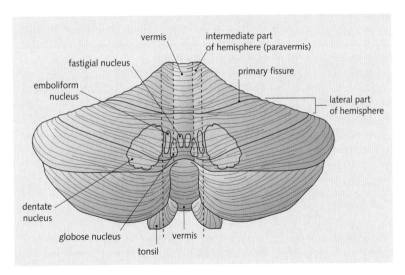

Fig. 5.15 Sagittal section through cerebellar cortex showing lobules and folia.

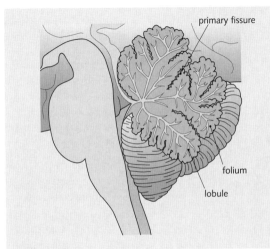

- Stellate and basket cells inhibit the Purkinje cells. The inhibition from Golgi, stellate, and basket cells helps to prevent submaximally stimulated Purkinje and granule cells from firing (reducing noise).

The output of the cerebellar cortex is provided by the Purkinje cells which form GABAergic (inhibitory) projections to the cerebellar nuclei, the cells of which then project to other parts of the central nervous system.

Functional units of the cerebellum

The vestibulocerebellum receives information from the vestibular nuclei (changes in head position relative to body position and gravity) and visual information indirectly from the lateral geniculate nuclei, superior colliculi, and visual cortex. It projects to the vestibular nuclei, which then link to

Inputs to the cerebellum				
Input from	**Tract**	**Peduncle**	**Termination**	**Processing**
Spinal cord	Spinocerebellar (anterior)	Superior	Vermis	Control of axial muscles, muscle tone
Medulla (gracile, cuneate + trigeminal nuclei)	Spinocerebellar (posterior)	Inferior	Paravermis	Distal limb coordination, muscle tone
Midbrain	Tectocerebellar	Inferior	Vermis	Visual + auditory
Olivary nucleus	Olivocerebellar (via medulla)	Inferior	Paravermis	Sensory
Vestibular nucleus	Vestibulocerebellar (via medulla)	Inferior	Vermis + floccus	Balance
Basilar pons	Pontocerebellar (via pons)	Middle	Lateral hemispheres	Motor planning

Fig. 5.16 Inputs to the cerebellum.

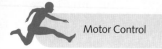

Fig. 5.17 Cerebellar outputs.

Cerebellar output			
Region	Via deep nucleus	Termination	Function
vermis	fastigial	motor cortex, reticular formation	control of axial muscles as movement progresses
paravermis	interposed	red nucleus—influencing fibers to thalamus and motor cortex, and those in rubrospinal tract	control of distal muscles as movement progresses
hemispheres	dentate	red nucleus and premotor cortex	movement planning, timing, and initiation
flocculonodular lobe	direct projection	lateral vestibular nucleus	control of balance and postural reflexes

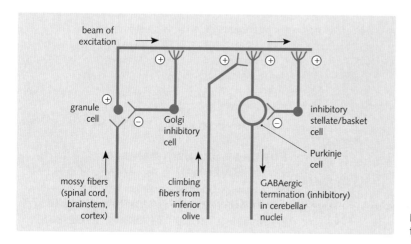

Fig. 5.18 The processing circuit in the cerebellar cortex.

the motor neurons innervating the extraocular muscles and those controlling axial (neck) muscles (balance) for the coordination of head and eye movements.

The spinocerebellum receives its main input from the spinocerebellar tract and is concerned with the control of postural muscle tone in axial and limb muscles (by setting γ-motor neuron output which affects α-motor neuron activity through the reflex loop) and influences movement execution.

• The vermal portion receives information from auditory, visual, and vestibular systems, and sensory information from the proximal body. It projects to the fastigial nucleus which influences the vestibulospinal and reticulospinal systems.

• The intermediate hemisphere receives sensory information from the distal body and projects through the globose and emboliform nuclei to primarily influence the red nucleus and the rubrospinal tract. It also projects to the contralateral motor cortex (via the thalamus).

The cerebrocerebellum controls precision in rapid and dextrous movements, receiving information from cortical motor and sensory areas via the basilar pontine nuclei and the massive pontocerebellar system of axons. The cerebrocerebellum is inserted in a processing loop that includes corticopontine and pontocerebellar connections, cerebellar nuclear projections from the cerebellar dentate nucleus to the ventrolateral thalamic nucleus, and thalamocortical connections.

Error detection in cerebellar movement control

The Purkinje cells exhibit a modification to their firing pattern when errors in planned movement occur. This change consists of "complex" spikes where, after the initial depolarization caused by Na^+ influx, there is a smaller continued depolarization (a "plateau") resulting from an influx of Ca^{2+}, and then additional spikes superimposed on the plateau, also due to the opening of Ca^{2+} channels. This pattern of firing is produced by a climbing fiber input and suggests that the olivocerebellar tract is involved in error detection.

When a new movement is performed, a large and long-lasting activation of Purkinje cells is sometimes observed. It is believed by some that this activity corresponds to error correction signals being stored in motor memory at a special type of modifiable synapse capable of long-term depression. As the movement is practiced, fewer errors are made and the Purkinje activation decreases.

Effects of cerebellar lesions

Cerebellar disease produces movement dysfunction in limbs ipsilateral to the lesion; volitional movements are still present although defective. Common signs of cerebellar dysfunction include:

- Ataxia—uncoordinated movements.
- Dysmetria—movemnets that overshoot or undershoot their intended target.
- Dysdiadochokinesia—an inability to perform rapid alternating movements.
- Intention tremor—appearance of a tremor when performing a voluntary movement (the opposite of resting tremor as seen in Parkinson's disease).

Lesions can result from head injury, tumors, hemorrhage, ischemia, and Friedreich's ataxia. The white matter pathways carrying the connections can be damaged in multiple sclerosis. Effects include the following:

- Disturbances of posture—wide-base standing position, ataxic gait, nystagmus in flocculonodular damage.
- Disturbances of muscle tone (hypotonia) and axial and truncal control—in vermis and intermediate hemisphere damage.
- Disturbances in control of precision movements—delays in starting and stopping movements,

tremor increasing in severity through a movement, disorders in movement timing so that movements become decomposed into their components, and poor coordination of muscle groups, making rapidly alternating movements very difficult.

The vestibular system, posture, and locomotion

Control of posture

Posture

Posture is the relative position of the trunk, head, and limbs in space. To keep posture stable, the body's center of gravity needs to be maintained in position over its support base.

Postural reflexes are required to correct changes caused by displacement of the center of gravity (by either external forces or deliberate movement). Postural change is detected by musculoskeletal proprioceptors, the vestibular apparatus, and the visual system.

The vestibular system

Fig. 5.19 shows the components of the vestibular system. A more complete diagram is included in Chapter 9 (Fig. 9.1). The vestibular apparatus detects changes in head position, linear acceleration, and angular acceleration. The vestibular nuclei use this information together with afferent nerves from neck muscles and cervical vertebrae to determine if the head is moving alone or if the head and body are both moving. The nuclei can influence antigravity and axial musculature via a direct projection into the spinal cord. The vestibular system also has outputs which affect eye movements.

The receptor system

The inner ear apparatus is contained within a number of interconnected membranous tunnels. These are cavities within the petrous temporal bone—the bony labyrinth—which contains fluid (perilymph). Within the bony labyrinth, and bathed in perilymph, is the membranous labyrinth which is filled with endolymph. Perilymph closely resembles cerebrospinal fluid, but endolymph is much more similar to intracellular fluid in terms of ion concentration.

Two "otolith organs"—the saccule and utricle—lie in the middle of the inner ear (the vestibule). Both of

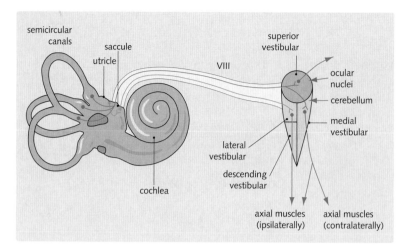

Fig. 5.19 The vestibular system.

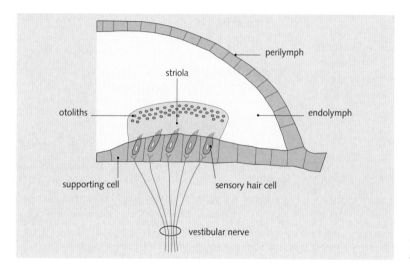

Fig. 5.20 Structure of the otolith organs.

these structures contain patches of hair cells called maculae (Fig. 5.20).

- The saccular macula is oriented vertically, and detects changes in linear acceleration in the vertical plane and changes in head position during lateral tilt.
- The utricular macula is oriented horizontally, and detects changes in linear acceleration in the horizontal plane and changes in head position during flexion and extension of the neck.

The semicircular canals are arranged at right angles to each other and, together, they detect angular acceleration in all three planes of three-dimensional space. Each canal has a swelling (ampulla) near its attachment to the utricle, which contains the hair

cells projecting from a ridge (crista) into a semiflexible, jelly-like substance (cupula) whose shape is influenced by endolymph movement (Fig. 5.21).

Head movement is detected by movement of the membranous labyrinth relative to the endolymph which, because of its viscosity and inertia, lags a little behind.

Specialized hair cells in the ampulla of each semicircular duct have projections from their apical surface (several stereocilia and a single kinocilium) into the jelly-like cupula that protrudes into the endolymph.

The cupula is deflected by endolymph movement and this moves the hair cell stereocilia. Since all the hair cell cilia in the ampulla of a single semicircular

Fig. 5.21 Structure of ampullar crista.

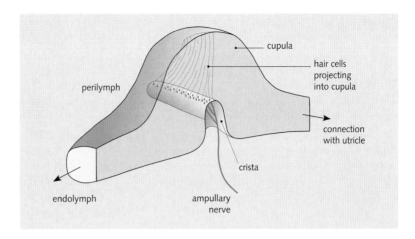

Fig. 5.22 Vestibular hair cells. Bending of the stereocilia toward the kinocilium causes ion channels to open and results in depolarization of the cell. The opposite happens when the stereocilia are bent the other way.

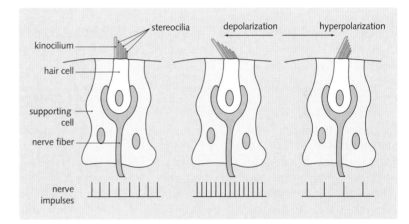

duct are similarly polarized, all the hair cells are excited by endolymph movement in one direction or all are inhibited by endolymph movement in the opposite direction, as shown in Fig. 5.22. Deflection of the cilia in a specific direction mechanically opens (depolarizes) or closes (hyperpolarizes) cation channels in the cilia membrane. If the stereocilia are deflected toward the kinocilium, the cell is depolarized and releases more transmitter. Conversely, the cell will be hyperpolarized if the stereocilia are deflected away from the kinocilium and will release less transmitter.

Improving the quality of postural information

Hair cells show greatest alteration in membrane permeability when the stereocilia are moved in one direction. To detect different degrees of tilt and different degrees of flexion, the hair cells in the maculae of the utricle and sacule are oriented in various planes so that they respond best to a particular head position. The vestibular nuclei can use this information to assess head position precisely.

Disturbances of the vestibular system (such as might be caused by infection in the middle ear) may lead to a false sense of rotational movement (vertigo), nausea, and eye movement problems. It is often caused by a disruption in endolymph flow due to the presence of debris in the semicircular ducts or the otolithic organs, and may be worse in particular head positions.

Complementary pathways

The brain receives complementary information from the two labyrinths since they are located on opposite sides of the head. For example, as the head turns, one set of hair cells becomes depolarized, whereas the

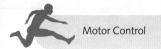

complementary set on the other side becomes hyperpolarized. This organization helps to mediate postural reflexes.

The vestibular nuclei

The vestibular nuclei lie in the medulla, on the floor of the fourth ventricle, and receive information from the hair cells through the vestibular nerve (VIII).

- The semicircular canals project to the superior and medial vestibular nuclei.
- The otolith organs project to the lateral vestibular nuclei.

The medial vestibulospinal tract projects bilaterally, and the lateral vestibulospinal tract projects ipsilaterally. Both tracts influence axial and limb extensor muscles. The vestibular nuclei also project to the thalamus, cerebellum, oculomotor nuclei, and contralateral vestibular nuclei. These connections are important in maintaining eye position in the presence of head rotation.

Responses to external and self-generated disturbances

External disturbance alters postural equilibrium. The vestibular system detects postural change and mediates postural adjustment. Together with the cerebellum, the vestibular system can adapt postural reflexes (e.g., responses on a moving platform, as shown in Fig. 5.23).

Responses to self-generated disturbance show that the vestibular system has a feedforward control mechanism. This is important for eye movements, as a change in head position will alter the the image on the retina. To stabilize the retinal image, the vestibular system detects head movements and drives compensatory eye movements. The circuit for this is shown in Fig. 5.24. The vestibulo-ocular reflex is an open loop reflex as it works without feedback. The cerebellum regulates the gain of the reflex (amount of eye movement to compensate for head movement). Eye movement control is discussed more fully in Chapter 8.

Vestibular and neck reflexes

The vestibular system mediates some of the neck reflexes (Fig. 5.25).

Control of locomotion

Locomotion requires a coordination of the systems controlling posture and the systems producing voluntary movement. This ensures that the body is supported against gravity and that the center of gravity lies over the support base during propulsion.

A rhythm of muscle activity is needed as each limb takes its turn in supporting the body and moving

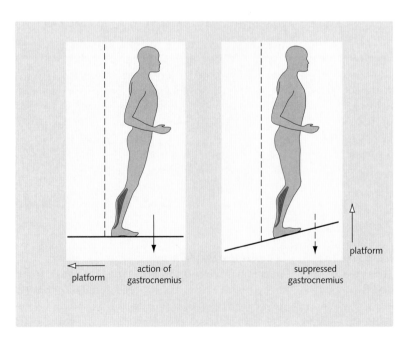

Fig. 5.23 Reflex responses to postural change can be altered.

Fig. 5.24 The horizontal vestibulo-ocular reflex.

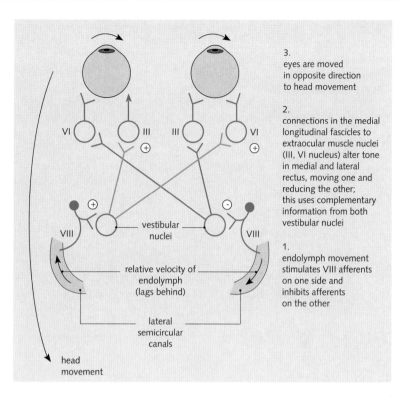

3.
eyes are moved in opposite direction to head movement

2.
connections in the medial longitudinal fascicles to extraocular muscle nuclei (III, VI nucleus) alter tone in medial and lateral rectus, moving one and reducing the other; this uses complementary information from both vestibular nuclei

1.
endolymph movement stimulates VIII afferents on one side and inhibits afferents on the other

VI   III   III   VI

vestibular nuclei

VIII   VIII

relative velocity of endolymph (lags behind)

lateral semicircular canals

head movement

Neck reflexes	
Reflex	**Action**
Vestibulocolic	Stabilizes the position of the head, e.g., if the body is tilted forward, it returns the head to the vertical position. Synergistic with the cervicocolic reflex of the neck musculature
Vestibulospinal	Tilting the head forward (e.g., when falling) causes extension of the upper limbs and flexion of the lower limbs. This protects from the impact of the fall. Antagonistic with the cervicospinal reflexes

Fig. 5.25 The vestibular neck reflexes. Note that these are overcome by cortical control in normal situations.

it forward. The circuits that generate this pattern of activity are in the spinal cord and can be activated by higher centres (e.g., the brainstem).

A network of interneurons in the spinal cord govern the activity of motor neurons; these are known as central pattern generators (CPGs). One CPG will activate flexor muscles, and another extensors, the two being mutually inhibitory.

Renshaw cells in the spinal cord inhibit interneurons that are firing. Therefore activation of CPG-1 will cause its own inactivation (via Renshaw cells), which then removes the inhibition of CPG-2. This rhythmic switching may be modified by 1b afferent information from the Golgi tendon organs which prevents excessive tension in either muscle group.

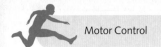

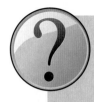

- Explain the difference between feedback and feedforward control with examples.
- What is a motor program? How is it learned?
- What is a motor unit? Explain the term innervation ratio with examples.
- Relate the structure of the muscle spindle to its function.
- Contrast the functions of the muscle spindle and the Golgi tendon organ.
- Draw a diagram illustrating the circuitry of the biceps reflex.
- Where is the primary motor cortex, and how is it organized?
- Relate the signs of an upper motor neuron lesion to pyramidal tract function and compare these with the signs of a lower motor neuron lesion.
- Contrast the direct and indirect pathways within the basal ganglia with regard to their structure and functions.
- What are the signs and symptoms of parkinsonism. What causes do you know?
- What are the functions of the cerebellum? Relate them to the effects of lesions.
- What are the functions of the otolith organs and semicircular canals? Relate this to their structure.
- How does the vestibular system contribute to the vestibulo-ocular reflex?
- Describe the basic control of locomotion.

6. The Brainstem

In this chapter, you will learn about:
- The anatomy of the brainstem, including the cranial nerve nuclei.
- The functions of the reticular formation.
- How sleep affects the electroencephalograph.

The brainstem nuclei

This section describes the anatomy of the brainstem by relating cross-sectional appearance to the overall structure of the brainstem. A knowledge of the functions of the cranial nerves is essential for understanding the basis for the tests that confirm brain death. The trochlear nerve (IV) is the only nerve to exit via the dorsal aspect of the brainstem. It has a tortuous intracranial course, and is particularly susceptible to damage following head trauma.

Fig. 6.1 demonstrates the location where the cranial nerves leave the brainstem and the levels of the seven brainstem sections are shown in Figs. 6.2 to 6.8.

Fig. 6.2 illustrates a cross-section of the caudal medulla oblongata just above its connection with the spinal cord. At this level, the right and left "pyramids" can be seen as enlargements of the anterior part of the medulla. This is where the motor fibers decussate before continuing down the spinal cord as the corticospinal tracts. The gracile and cuneate sensory nuclei are found posteriorly at this level, while the spinal trigeminal nucleus (cranial nerve V) is positioned posterolaterally.

Fig. 6.3 illustrates a cross-section through the middle of the medulla at a level through the decussation of the medial lemnisci. This represents the formation of the medial lemniscus of one side by the crossing of sensory (internal arcuate) fibers originating from cell bodies in the contralateral gracile and cuneate nuclei. The spinal trigeminal tracts and nuclei, hypoglossal nuclei, and dorsal motor nuclei of the vagus can also be seen at this level.

Elevated intracranial pressure can cause the medulla and cerebellar tonsils to herniate downward toward the foramen magnum. Symptoms may include headache, neck stiffness, and paralysis of cranial nerves IX–XII. Lumbar puncture is very dangerous in these patients as it may lead to further herniation of the brain through the foramen magnum, and ischemia of the compressed areas. The latter process is often referred to as "coning."

The rostral medulla (Fig. 6.4) forms the floor of the fourth ventricle. There is a much larger volume of gray matter at this level, as demonstrated by the increased number of nuclei here. The reticular formation is found in the core region of the medulla, anterior to the cranial nerve nuclei and lateral to the medial longitudinal fasciculus and medial lemniscus. The pyramids contain descending corticofugal fibers including corticospinal and a few corticobulbar fibers and are located on the anterior surface of the medulla.

Fig. 6.5 shows a cross-section through the caudal pons. The medial lemniscus can still be seen, but has rotated by 90° to lie transversely, separating the pontine tegmentum posteriorly from the basilar pontine gray anteriorly. The medial longitudinal fasciculus lies just beneath the floor of the fourth ventricle, and is the pathway connecting the vestibular nuclei with the nuclei controlling eye movements, the abducens, trochlear, and oculomotor nuclei.

The mid- to rostral portion of the pons (Fig. 6.6) is similar to the caudal levels but, in addition, contains the motor and principal sensory nuclei of the trigeminal nerve (V). The middle cerebellar peduncle (brachium pontis) is entering the cerebellum and is primarily composed of the axons of

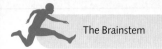

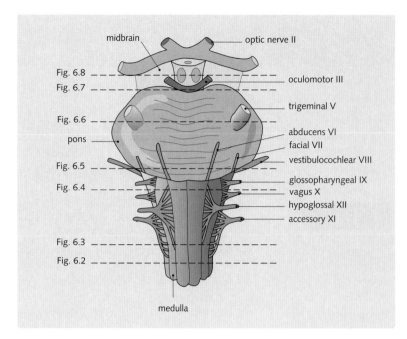

Fig. 6.1 Cranial nerves as they leave the brainstem.

midbrain

optic nerve II

Fig. 6.8

Fig. 6.7

oculomotor III

trigeminal V

Fig. 6.6

pons

abducens VI

facial VII

vestibulocochlear VIII

Fig. 6.5

Fig. 6.4

glossopharyngeal IX

vagus X

hypoglossal XII

accessory XI

Fig. 6.3

Fig. 6.2

medulla

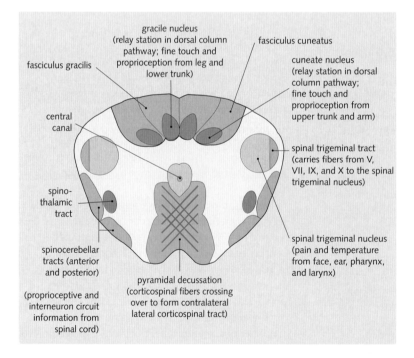

gracile nucleus
(relay station in dorsal column pathway; fine touch and proprioception from leg and lower trunk)

fasciculus cuneatus

fasciculus gracilis

cuneate nucleus
(relay station in dorsal column pathway; fine touch and proprioception from upper trunk and arm)

central canal

spinal trigeminal tract
(carries fibers from V, VII, IX, and X to the spinal trigeminal nucleus)

spino-thalamic tract

spinocerebellar tracts (anterior and posterior)

(proprioceptive and interneuron circuit information from spinal cord)

pyramidal decussation
(corticospinal fibers crossing over to form contralateral lateral corticospinal tract)

spinal trigeminal nucleus
(pain and temperature from face, ear, pharynx, and larynx)

Fig. 6.2 Section through lower medulla (level of motor decussation).

Fig. 6.3 Section through mid-medulla (level of sensory decussation).

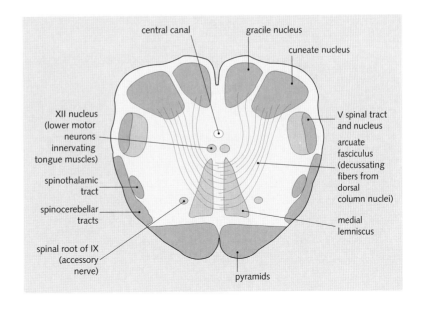

central canal

gracile nucleus

cuneate nucleus

XII nucleus (lower motor neurons innervating tongue muscles)

V spinal tract and nucleus

arcuate fasciculus (decussating fibers from dorsal column nuclei)

spinothalamic tract

spinocerebellar tracts

medial lemniscus

spinal root of IX (accessory nerve)

pyramids

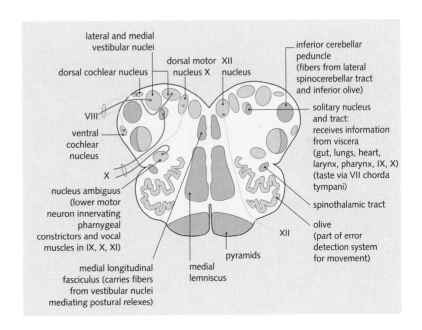

lateral and medial vestibular nuclei

dorsal cochlear nucleus

dorsal motor nucleus X

XII nucleus

inferior cerebellar peduncle (fibers from lateral spinocerebellar tract and inferior olive)

VIII

solitary nucleus and tract: receives information from viscera (gut, lungs, heart, larynx, pharynx, IX, X) (taste via VII chorda tympani)

ventral cochlear nucleus

X

spinothalamic tract

nucleus ambiguus (lower motor neuron innervating pharnygeal constrictors and vocal muscles in IX, X, XI)

olive (part of error detection system for movement)

XII

medial longitudinal fasciculus (carries fibers from vestibular nuclei mediating postural relexes)

medial lemniscus

pyramids

Fig. 6.4 Section through upper medulla (level of inferior olive).

81

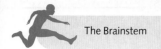

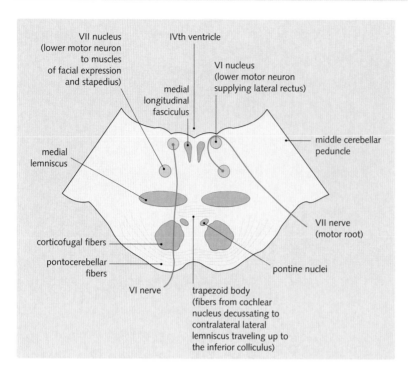

Fig. 6.5 Section through lower pons (level of the facial colliculus). Superior cerebellar peduncle and vestibular nucleus not shown.

In the figure (Fig. 6.5):
- VII nucleus (lower motor neuron to muscles of facial expression and stapedius)
- IVth ventricle
- VI nucleus (lower motor neuron supplying lateral rectus)
- medial longitudinal fasciculus
- middle cerebellar peduncle
- medial lemniscus
- VII nerve (motor root)
- corticofugal fibers
- pontocerebellar fibers
- pontine nuclei
- VI nerve
- trapezoid body (fibers from cochlear nucleus decussating to contralateral lateral lemniscus traveling up to the inferior colliculus)

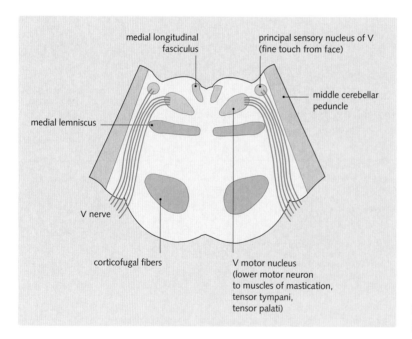

In the figure (Fig. 6.6):
- medial longitudinal fasciculus
- principal sensory nucleus of V (fine touch from face)
- middle cerebellar peduncle
- medial lemniscus
- V nerve
- corticofugal fibers
- V motor nucleus (lower motor neuron to muscles of mastication, tensor tympani, tensor palati)

Fig. 6.6 Section through upper pons (level of the trigeminal nuclei).

Fig. 6.7 Section through lower midbrain (level of inferior colliculus).

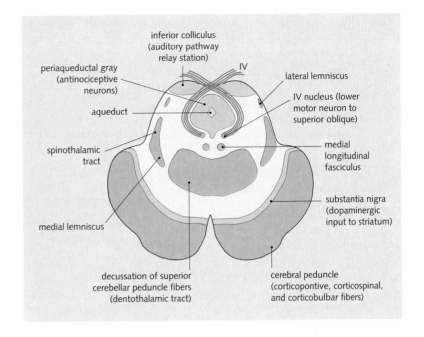

inferior colliculus (auditory pathway relay station)

IV

periaqueductal gray (antinociceptive neurons)

lateral lemniscus

IV nucleus (lower motor neuron to superior oblique)

aqueduct

medial longitudinal fasciculus

spinothalamic tract

substantia nigra (dopaminergic input to striatum)

medial lemniscus

decussation of superior cerebellar peduncle fibers (dentothalamic tract)

cerebral peduncle (corticopontive, corticospinal, and corticobulbar fibers)

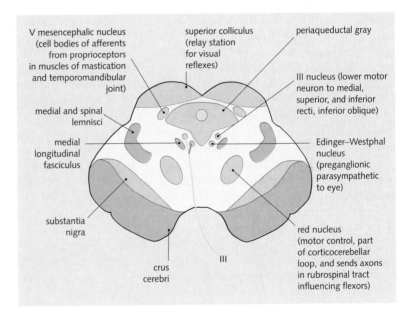

V mesencephalic nucleus (cell bodies of afferents from proprioceptors in muscles of mastication and temporomandibular joint)

superior colliculus (relay station for visual reflexes)

periaqueductal gray

III nucleus (lower motor neuron to medial, superior, and inferior recti, inferior oblique)

medial and spinal lemnisci

medial longitudinal fasciculus

Edinger–Westphal nucleus (preganglionic parasympathetic to eye)

substantia nigra

crus cerebri

III

red nucleus (motor control, part of corticocerebellar loop, and sends axons in rubrospinal tract influencing flexors)

Fig. 6.8 Section through upper midbrain (level of superior colliculus).

neurons in the contralateral basilar pontine nuclei which receive a massive input from the cerebral cortex.

The anterolateral aspect of the midbrain is made up of two large descending bundles of corticofugal fibers, the crura cerebri (singular, crus cerebri), which comprise a portion of the cerebral peduncle (Fig. 6.7). Through each of these runs a darkly (black) pigmented area—the substantia nigra. The cerebral aqueduct connects the third ventricle to the more caudal fourth ventricle. Just posterior to the aqueduct lies the tectum, which comprises the superior and inferior colliculi (Fig. 6.8). This region is also referred to as the quadrigeminal plate.

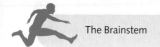

The cerebral aqueduct in the midbrain is extremely narrow and vulnerable to blockage by tumors. This type of occlusion causes noncommunicating hydrocephalus.

The reticular formation

Location and organization

If all the nuclei and tracts are identified in the brainstem (medulla, pons, and midbrain), a central core of cells and fibers remains. These are loosely arranged as a network and are referred to as the brainstem reticular formation. The largest of the cell bodies tend to be located ventromedially, while the smaller cell bodies are aggregated dorsolaterally. It is likely that these cells represent a rostral extension of spinal cord interneurons. Adjacent to either side of the midline lie the raphe nuclei.

In the reticular formation, cell groupings can be identified on the basis of the specific neurotransmitter contained within the cells. These are noradrenaline, 5-hydroxytryptamine (5-HT, serotonin), acetylcholine, and dopamine. The projections of these cells are particularly widespread in the CNS, perhaps with the exception of the dopaminergic system which projects in a more restricted fashion to the neostriatum, limbic areas, prefrontal cortex, and anterior cingulate cortex.

Some of the reticular core is not yet defined in terms of neurotransmitter content but can be partially defined according to function.
- A sensory portion in the caudal medulla and caudal pons (receiving spinoreticular fibers).
- A motor portion in the rostral medulla and rostral pons that receives collaterals from the bundle of descending corticofugal fibers and gives rise to the reticulospinal tracts.

Cells in the pontine and medullary reticular formation project rostrally to the midbrain reticular formation, which in turn projects mainly to the hypothalamus and also the thalamic reticular nuclei and the intralaminar nuclei. There is also a substantial descending projection from the hypothalamus and prefrontal association cortex into the reticular formation.

The cells of the reticular formation can be histologically separated from other neurons in that:
- They have large, transversely (or mediolaterally) oriented dendritic trees that receive information from many ascending and descending fiber systems.
- They project diffusely either to rostral parts of the nervous system or to the spinal cord, with many reticular cells having both rostrally and caudally directed axonal collaterals.

Functions of the reticular formation

The functions of the reticular formation include:
- Sleeping and waking—some parts of the reticular formation are involved in producing sleep states and others in awakening mechanisms via their projections to the thalamus and prefrontal cortex. This is related to behavioral arousal and awareness, and is thought to be mainly due to activity in the noradrenergic system. These ascending reticular projections form the basis of the reticular activating system.
- Modulation of sensory information directed to the thalamic relay nuclei. This includes the modulation of pain—the reticular system may have a role in the "gating" mechanism.
- Motor control via descending raphe projections to spinal interneurons and transmitting information from lateral parts of the reticular formation to the cerebellum.
- Modulation of respiration.
- Modulation of the responsiveness of hippocampal neurons.
- Integration of autonomic functions, particularly cardiovascular. In sleep, heart rate, blood pressure, and respiration all decline; before awakening, they are adjusted so that the transition from horizontal to vertical does not cause fainting.
- Control of endocrine functions via the hypothalamic nuclei.
- Possible role in cognition.
- Motor acts involving motivation and reward (dopaminergic system, particularly the mesolimbic projections from the midbrain to the ventral striatum).

Fig. 7.2 Spinal cord efferents to the sympathetic chain.

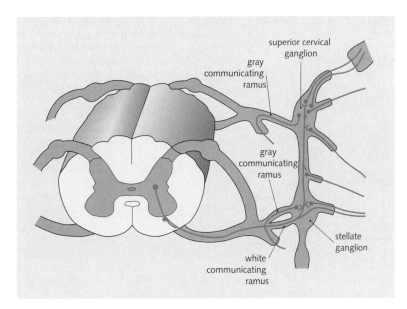

the "postganglionic" neurons. Postganglionic axons are unmyelinated and reach their peripheral target sites by a variety of strategies. For the head and neck, they form a plexus around the carotid arteries and gain access to the interior of the skull by the internal carotid artery.

Afferent fibers course from the periphery toward the CNS and pass through the paravertebral and prevertebral ganglia without synapsing, reaching their cell bodies in the dorsal root ganglia. From here the central process enters the spinal cord via the dorsal root and terminates within the dorsal horn gray matter.

Exceptions to the general pattern of sympathetic nervous system innervation

Some preganglionic fibers do not synapse in the pre- or paravertebral ganglia, but carry on to ganglia closer to their target organs via the splanchnic nerves (thoracic, lumbar, or sacral). The celiac, aorticorenal, superior mesenteric, and inferior mesenteric ganglia contain cell bodies providing the postganglionic sympathetic nervous system innervation to the gut, kidney, liver, pancreas, and urogenital organs. Some preganglionic fibers continue to the adrenal medulla. Here, they are responsible for the glandular secretion of catecholamines from cells that are functionally similar to postganglionic sympathetic neurons.

The adrenal medulla receives a direct innervation from the spinal cord that is not interrupted by a synapse in a ganglion.

Neurotransmission in the sympathetic nervous system

The transmitter released by preganglionic neurons at the ganglia (and also those synapsing in the adrenal medulla) is acetylcholine, which binds to postsynaptic nicotinic receptors. The nicotinic receptor is a cation channel which, when opened, produces a fast excitatory postsynaptic potential. The transmitter released by postganglionic neurons is noradrenaline, except in certain sweat glands where acetylcholine is released and binds to muscarinic receptors (which are slower metabotropic receptors).

Transmission occurs at specialized structures along the length of the postganglionic axon called varicosities, which synthesize, release, take up, and metabolize noradrenaline. This process is called "en passage" transmission, as the action potential does not end when noradrenaline is released but continues on to the next varicosity.

Cells of the adrenal medulla release noradrenaline and adrenaline into the circulation, permitting the sympathetic nervous system to have a general humoral action on adrenergic receptors in the body.

The effect of noradrenaline release is dependent on the type of receptor that is present in the target organ, as shown in Fig. 7.3.

Other transmitters

Often, cotransmitters are released with the main transmitter in the sympathetic nervous system to

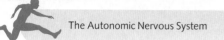
Adrenergic receptors			
Adrenergic receptor	Location	Second messenger	Function
α_1	smooth muscle in blood vessels and dilator pupillae	IP_3	contraction
α_2	smooth muscle in blood vessels, presynaptically on adrenergic synapses	decreased cAMP	contraction, reduced transmitter release
β_1	heart muscle, presynaptically on adrenergic synapses	increased cAMP	increased heart rate and force of contraction, increased transmitter release
β_2	smooth muscle in blood vessels and bronchi	decreased cAMP	relaxation

Fig. 7.3 Adrenergic receptors: location, second messenger, and function.

give a longer-lasting and more subtle modulatory influence on postsynaptic activity (e.g., ATP is released along with noradrenaline at postganglionic sympathetic nerve endings).

Drugs acting on the sympathetic nervous system
The ganglia
Drugs affecting ganglionic transmission have no clinical use. They have complex actions because parasympathetic and sympathetic postganglionic neurons are influenced at the same time, often with opposing effects. Agonists at ganglionic acetylcholine receptors (e.g., nicotine) produce hypertension and tachycardia. Antagonists (e.g., hexamethonium) produce hypotension, but cannot be used as antihypertensive agents because of their side-effect profile.

Although nicotine initially stimulates neurons in the ganglia, subsequently it causes a depolarization block when made available in high concentrations. This causes hypotension and decreased gut motility.

Target organs
Noradrenergic transmission can be altered by interfering with noradrenaline synthesis, release, or postsynaptic interaction with different receptor subtypes. Drugs used clinically are shown in Fig. 7.4.

Structure and function of the parasympathetic nervous system

Physiological role of the parasympathetic nervous system
The parasympathetic nervous system has many actions, which can be described as:
- Opposing some effects of the sympathetic nervous system (increasing heart rate, gut motility, and bronchiolar diameter).
- Controlling body functions under nonstressful conditions, working either alone or with the sympathetic nervous system (e.g., ciliary muscle for accommodation for near objects; gastrointestinal secretions; secretions of the nose, mouth, and eye; micturition; defecation; sexual function).

The functions of the parasympathetic system can be broadly summarized as "rest and digest."

Structure of the parasympathetic nervous system
There are two clusters of preganglionic neurons at either end of the spinal cord (Fig. 7.5).

90

Fig. 7.4 Drugs acting on the sympathetic nervous system.

Drugs acting on the sympathetic nervous system			
Drug	**Action**	**Clinical use**	**Side effects**
adrenaline	α, β agonist	anaphylaxis, cardiac arrest	hypertension, dysrhythmia
salbutamol	β_2 agonist	asthma	tachycardia, dysrhythmia, tremor
clonidine	partial α_2 agonist	hypertension	drowsiness, postural hypotension
prazosin	α_1 antagonist	hypertension	hypotension, tachycardia, impotence
atenolol	β_1 antagonist	hypertension, acute coronary, syndromes, tachyarrhythmias	heart failure, fatigue, cold extremities, less bronchoconstriction than nonselective β antagonists

The cranial parasympathetic nervous system outflow comes from several nuclei in the brainstem. Structures in the head are supplied by the ciliary, pterygopalatine, otic, and submandibular ganglia which receive inputs from cranial nerves III, VII, and IX. Organs in the thorax and abdomen receive their parasympathetic supply via the vagus (Xth) nerve, which links with (synapses in) diffusely distributed collections of postganglionic neurons in the walls of, or close to, the target organs.

The sacral parasympathetic nervous system outflow comes from preganglionic neurons whose cell bodies lie in a column in the ventral horn running from segments S2 to S4 of the spinal cord. Their axons leave the cord through the ventral root, the spinal nerve, and then continue in the anterior primary ramus. They enter a branch of the anterior primary ramus called a pelvic splanchnic nerve. The latter nerves course to the inferior mesenteric or hypogastric plexus where they pass straight through to reach postganglionic parasympathetic neurons located near or within the walls of their target organs in the hindgut or pelvis.

Neurotransmission in the parasympathetic nervous system

As in the sympathetic nervous system, preganglionic parasympathetic neurons release acetylcholine onto nicotinic receptors associated with postganglionic neurons.

At target organs, postganglionic neurons release acetylcholine onto muscarinic receptors, which show subtype variation localized to different target organs (Fig. 7.6).

Drugs acting on the parasympathetic nervous system

The drugs in clinical use that affect the function of the parasympathetic nervous system interact with the receptors on the target organs (Fig. 7.7).

The enteric nervous system

The enteric nervous system is a neural system embedded in the wall of the gastrointestinal tract, pancreas, and gall bladder. It consists of two tubular systems:

• The submucosal (Meissner's) plexus, which lies between the mucous membrane and the circular layer of smooth muscle.
• The myenteric (Auerbach's) plexus, which lies between the inner circular and outer longitudinal smooth muscle layers.

In Hirschsprung's disease, there is a congenital absence of Auerbach's plexus in the midportion of the colon. This prevents normal peristalsis in that region and leads to distension of that portion of the colon (megacolon) as fecal matter gradually accumulates since it cannot be moved further distally in the colon.

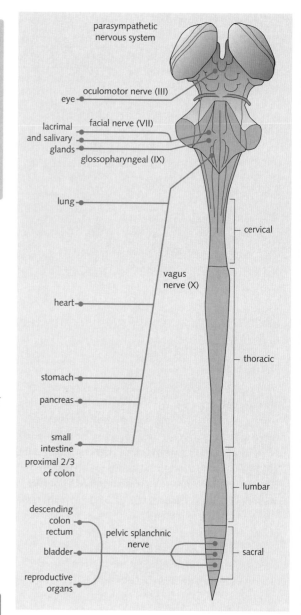

Fig. 7.5 Organization of the parasympathetic nervous system.

Each system contains both sensory and motor modalities. Each system receives inputs from other parts of the autonomic nervous system but also each has intrinsic activity that allows it to function independently of the autonomic system.

- The intrinsic sensory neurons monitor the mechanical state of the alimentary canal, the chemical status of the stomach and intestinal contents, and the hormonal levels in the portal blood vessels.
- The intrinsic motor neurons stimulate gut motility and secretions, as well as the diameter of local blood vessels.
- An extensive population of inhibitory and excitatory interneurons serves local reflex activity and joins rostrally and caudally adjacent segments of the gut tube.

The parasympathetic and sympathetic nervous systems can override the activity of the enteric division.

Disorders of the autonomic nervous system

Loss of the sympathetic innervation to the face causes Horner's syndrome. This is characterized by:
- Ptosis (drooping of the eyelid).
- Miosis (pupillary constriction).
- Anhydrosis (loss of sweating).
- Enophthalmos (eyes appear withdrawn into the orbit).

The innervation may be interrupted anywhere along its course—linkage between the hypothalamus and nuclei in the brainstem and cervical spinal cord are

rare sites of "central Horner's syndrome." Classically, compression of the stellate ganglion may occur in the presence of a carcinoma in the apex of the lung (Pancoast's tumor). Injury can also occur as the sympathetic fibers gain access to the head wrapped around the internal carotid artery (e.g., after dissection of the artery).

Fig. 7.6 Muscarinic receptors.

Muscarinic receptors		
Muscarinic subtype	**Location**	**Function**
M$_1$	Gastric parietal cells, enteric nervous system	Slow excitation of ganglia. Gastric acid secretion, gastrointestinal motility
M$_2$	Cardiac atrium	Vagal inhibition of heart. Decreased heart rate and force of contraction
M$_3$	Smooth muscle, glands	Secretion, contraction of smooth muscle, vascular relaxation

Drugs acting on the parasympathetic nervous system			
Drug	**Action**	**Use**	**Side effects**
pilocarpine	Partial muscarinic agonist	glaucoma (increased intraocular pressure), where increased constrictor pupillae action allows greater drainage of aqueous humor	cardiac slowing, increased gastrointestinal tract activity causing abdominal pain
atropine	Muscarinic antagonist	cardiac arrest, sinus bradycardia after myocardial infarction	dry mouth, dilated pupil, blurred vision, bronchodilatation, urinary retention
ipratropium	Muscarinic antagonist	asthma, causing bronchodilatation and inhibiting increases in mucous secretion	inhaled and does not pass easily into the circulation, so few side effects
dicyclomine	M$_1$ antagonist has direct relaxant effect on smooth muscle	reduce spasmodic activity of gastrointestinal tract in irritable bowel syndrome	less severe than atropine

Fig. 7.7 Drugs acting on the parasympathetic nervous system.

Section of the sympathetic trunk disrupts the control of structures innervated by that spinal level. Surgical section of sympathetic nerves in the cervicothoracic region has been used (with little success) to treat Raynaud's syndrome (where vasoconstriction causes painfully cold hands). A poorly understood feature of peripheral sympathetic injury is "reflex sympathetic dystrophy," which includes chronic pain, accompanied by dry, shiny, red skin and poor wound healing. When this condition can be localized to a particular nerve root, it is called "causalgia."

The effects of disrupting parasympathetic innervation are specific to the location of the lesion.

- A neurosyphilitic lesion in the oculomotor nerve causes loss of the pupillary light reflex, including dilatation of the pupil, but interestingly the accommodation reflex (the Argyll Robertson pupil) is preserved.
- Controlled ablation of a highly selective part of the vagal innervation to the stomach may be used as a treatment for excessive gastric acid secretion.
- Damage to the parasympathetic preganglionic fibers in the cauda equina causes loss of bladder control and sphincter dysfunction.

Pheochromocytomas, tumors of chromaffin tissue, are generally found in the adrenal medulla and secrete vast quantities of catecholamines. This causes hypertension (which may be extremely severe—with headaches and even intracranial hemorrhage as presenting features). A combination of alpha- and beta-adrenoceptor blockade is required until surgical removal is possible.

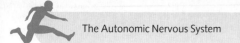

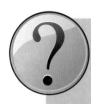

- What are the functions of the sympathetic nervous system?
- What drugs can modify sympathetic function, and how are they used?
- Relate the structure of the parasympathetic nervous system to its function.
- Compare the sympathetic and parasympathetic nervous systems. Explain why they are not exactly opposite in terms of function (give examples).
- How can drugs modulate parasympathetic function? In what clinical scenarios might they be used?
- Describe the structure and function of the enteric nervous system.

8. Vision

In this chapter, you will learn about:
- The macro- and microscopic anatomy of the eye.
- Retinal structure and function.
- Central visual pathways.
- Mechanisms of attention.
- Loss of vision.

The eye

Anatomy of the eye—transparent structures

The structures inside the eye are shown in Fig. 8.1.

The cornea is the transparent outer coat covering the pupil. It is continuous with the sclera (white of the eye) and consists of five layers. From the exterior inward they are:

- An epithelial layer of stratified squamous cells, which is richly innervated with sensory nerves and continuously bathed in tear fluid.
- The basement membrane that gives strength to the cornea.
- The corneal stroma occupies 90% of the thickness of the cornea. It consists of thin sheets of collagen fibrils that are oriented parallel to each other in the same sheet and at right angles to fibrils in sheets on either side. The spacing and arrangement of the fibrils gives the cornea its transparency.
- A basal lamina lines the inner surface of the stroma.
- The endothelial layer is a single layer of squamous cells, providing mechanisms for metabolic exchange between the aqueous humor and the cornea. It regulates the water content of the corneal stroma, preventing edema and consequent opacity.

The iris is the part of the eye that regulates how much light enters the eyeball. It is a pigmented, muscular structure that overlies the lens.

The lens is seen in the central space in the iris (the pupil). It appears black as it is transparent, and the choroid is visible. The lens consists of three parts:

- It is encapsulated in a basement membrane that is elastic, and strongest at the insertion of the suspensory ligament around the equator of the lens.

- Lining the inside of the capsule on its anterior surface is a layer of cuboidal cells (subcapsular epithelium). Epithelial cells near the lateral equator differentiate into lens fibers.
- Lens fibers are thin, flattened, and devoid of organelles and nuclei. They become filled with proteins (crystallins) and extend toward the center of the lens, producing a very dense central section.

The ciliary muscle contracts and relaxes the suspensory ligaments of the lens and, due to the intrinsic elasticity of the lens, it becomes more spherical. The increased curvature of the anterior surface of the lens changes its refractive power and this enables the lens to focus on an object relatively close to the eye (near vision). This represents the basis of the accommodation reflex.

The lens composition changes with age and it loses its intrinsic elasticity and thus its ability to accommodate. The lens also loses its transparency because of changes in the lens proteins. The opacities that develop in the lens are known as cataracts.

The shape of the eye is maintained by the tough sclera and an internal pressure (the intraocular pressure) exerted by the aqueous humor. The latter substance is produced by the ciliary epithelium, and flows into the posterior chamber, through the pupil, and into the anterior chamber. It passes out of the anterior chamber through the trabecular meshwork (a network of bands of tissue defining the edge of the anterior chamber) and the canal of Schlemm into the episcleral veins. The normal intraocular pressure is approximately 10–20 mmHg. If it exceeds 22 mmHg, the condition of glaucoma results and this can produce blindness by compressing the blood supply to the optic nerve. Blockage of the trabecular meshwork (e.g., by drugs that dilate the pupil, thereby pushing the iris up against the lens) can cause a sharp elevation in intraocular pressure and produce glaucoma. Such drugs should obviously be avoided in this condition.

The vitreous humor fills the posterior part of the eyeball. It is more viscous than the aqueous humor.

The eye is adapted for acute vision in that one small area of its sensory layer, the fovea, contains an

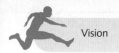

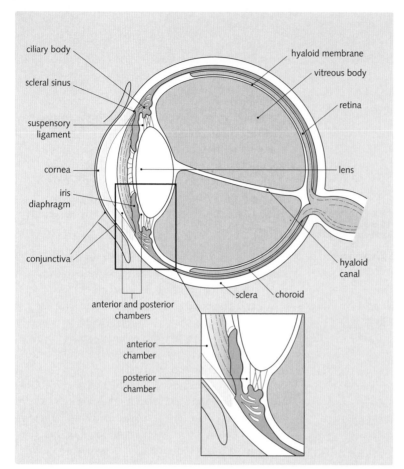

Fig. 8.1 Cross-section through the eye showing the main structures.

extremely high density of photoreceptors (cone photoreceptors for color vision in good illumination), which it can direct accurately and quickly to different areas of space.

This central area, the fovea, lies 3 mm lateral to the optic disk, as shown in Fig. 8.2, and it differs from the rest of the retina because:

- Only cone (wavelength-specific) receptors are present at a very high density.
- It has no overlying vascular network.
- Overlying nerve cell bodies are displaced to allow maximal light access.

The fovea is the central part of a small circular region called the macula lutea. On examination with an ophthalmoscope, the pigmented macula is semitransparent and the epithelium underlying the macula shows through, giving it a darker appearance than the rest of the retina. The visual axis of the eye does not correspond to its geometrical axis but rather

is displaced so that the visual axis runs through the fovea (Fig. 8.3).

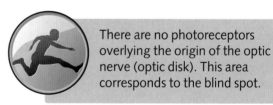

There are no photoreceptors overlying the origin of the optic nerve (optic disk). This area corresponds to the blind spot.

Optics of the eye

Light from a point of visual fixation is bent (refracted) so that a clearly focused image appears on the retina (Fig. 8.4). The lens for the visual system is a compound lens with interfaces of different refractive power (measured in diopters, D). These occur at the cornea:

- Between the anterior chamber and the lens.
- Between the lens and the vitreous body.

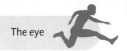

Fig. 8.2 Section of retina containing the fundus.

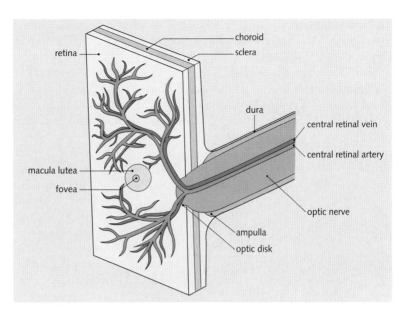

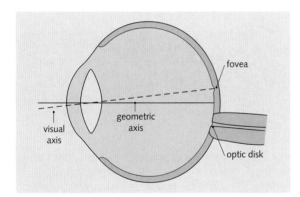

Fig. 8.3 Visual axis of the eye.

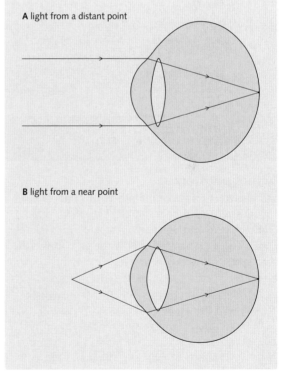

The total refractive power is 58.6 D, with most of the power (42 D) at the air–cornea interface.

Accommodation

As an individual refocuses from a distant to a near object, a sequence of three actions takes place. The two eyes converge in response to bilateral activation of the medial rectus muscles via the oculomotor nerve. At the same time, parasympathetic fibers activate the sphincter pupillae and ciliary muscles to bring about constriction of the pupil and change the shape of the lens. When the ciliary muscle contracts, it moves downward and forward. This reduces the tension in the radially arranged suspensory ligaments

Fig. 8.4 To change from distant to near vision the refractive power of the lens has to increase by around 3.3 diopters. For near vision the lens becomes better by a process termed accommodation.

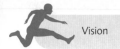

and allows the elastic lens to become more round (spheroidal). This alters the refractive power of the lens and focuses light from near targets (which reaches the surface of the eye as divergent rays) by convergence onto the retina. The lens is an elastic structure in young people, but it gradually hardens with age, loses its inherent elasticity, and can no longer readily change shape. As a consequence, near vision becomes impaired with increasing age, a phenomenon called presbyopia.

> The accommodation reflex comes into play when the eye is focused on a distant object and then is refocused on a near object. The two eyes converge, the pupils constrict, and the lens becomes more spherical. This reflex involves coordinated activity in the optic nerves, bilateral activation of the medial rectus skeletal muscles via the oculomotor nerves, and contraction of the sphincter pupillae and ciliary smooth muscles by parasympathetic fibers in the oculomotor nerves.

Retinal function and image processing

Visual pigments

Visual pigments within photoreceptors undergo a chemical change after absorbing the energy from photons, enabling transduction of light into a neural signal. The pigments used by the rod system and the cone system differ, reflecting their different functions.

Visual pigments have a characteristic structure consisting of the vitamin A aldehyde, retinal, covalently attached to a protein (one of the opsins). The second-messenger system modulated by the opsins involves cyclic guanosine monophosphate, cGMP (opsins resemble G-protein-coupled receptors).

The receptor function of the retina is carried out by two types of cells:
- Rods are very sensitive to light, respond best in dim light conditions (scotopic vision), and are found peripherally in the retina.

- Cones are less sensitive to light and respond best in bright light (photopic vision). There are three types of cones that respond to different wavelengths of light. Combinations of inputs from these receptors encode different colors. Cones are clustered in the fovea, where the high density leads to greater acuity.

In rods, the pigment is rhodopsin. Rhodopsin lies in the membrane of intracytoplasmic disks in the rod. It has seven membrane-spanning domains arranged around the retinal molecule, which attaches to the seventh transmembrane domain.

In cones, the variation in pigment is produced by different forms of opsin with their own specific interaction with retinal. This results in the different absorption sensitivities in the cone system:
- B cones at 420 nm (blue).
- G cones at 531 nm (green).
- R cones at 558 nm (red).

> Alterations in the photopigment within cone receptors lead to color blindness.

> The cornea and lens become yellow with age and this filters out much of the light in the blue wavelength band.

The retina responds to a restricted range of wavelengths of light. We see and perceive colors in the range 400 nm (violet) to 780 nm (red). Wavelengths either side of this range (as low as 400 nm and as high as 1400 nm) penetrate the eye, but have no receptors specialized for their detection. The activation cascade for signaling that light has reached the rod or cone outer segment, shown in Fig. 8.5, begins with the change in retinal and ends with an alteration in membrane permeability to cations.

The photosensitive part of rhodopsin is retinal, which changes its configuration when bombarded by photons (from 11-*cis*-retinal; with the terminal

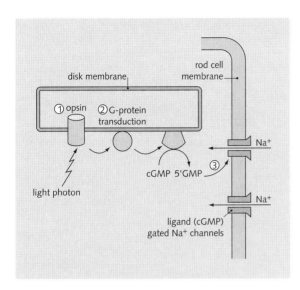

Fig. 8.5 Signal transduction of light impulses. (1) Conformational change. Afterward, all-*trans*-retinal no longer binds, which affects the G-protein transduction. (2) Increased activity of cGMP phosphodiesterase, which hydrolyzes cGMP, reducing its intracellular level. (3) Low cGMP levels close the ligand-gated channels, and thereby hyperpolarize the rod.

aldehyde group at an angle to the remainder of the molecule to all-*trans*-retinal; with the terminal aldehyde group in line with the remainder of the molecule). This disrupts the binding of retinal to opsin, causing the two to separate, producing a conformational change in opsin. This leads to a reduction in intracellular cGMP.

In darkness the cGMP-gated channels in the outer segment membrane are open because there has been no photon-induced reduction in the intracellular level of cGMP. The steady inflow of Na^+ (the "dark current") in the absence of light maintains the resting (depolarized) membrane of the receptor at −40 mV, producing a constant release of the neurotransmitter glutamate at its synapse.

After a reduction in cGMP as a result of photon activation of the visual pigment, the channels close, hyperpolarizing the cell and reducing glutamate release at the synapse. Greater light intensities produce greater hyperpolarization (up to a maximum of −70 mV with all the Na^+ channels closed).

Structure of the retina
The neural part of the retina responds to light, processes light signals from photoreceptors, and sends visual information to the thalamus and brainstem. The functions of different neurons in the retina depend on their connections and all the neural elements are supported by a particular type of glial cell, Müller's cell.

There is a blood–retina barrier at the endothelium of the capillary network formed by branches of the central retinal artery, on the anterior surface of the retina, and at the endothelium of the capillary network in the choroid.

The photoreceptors are situated in the most posterior layer of the retina. This means that light has to travel through several cell layers before reaching them. This is particularly true in the peripheral areas of the retina.

Rods and cones have different structures, as shown in Figs. 8.6 and 8.7, but share the following features:
- Outer segments, which contact the pigmented epithelial layer of the retina, contain highly folded membrane structures with visual pigments.
- Inner segments contain the nucleus and organelles.
- A synaptic terminal (the most anterior structure).

Fig. 8.8 compares the connections and functions of rods and cones.

Connections in the retina
Fig. 8.9 shows the circuit in the retina. Photoreceptor activity can evoke either excitatory or inhibitory responses in bipolar cells, depending on the type of postsynaptic glutamate receptor on the bipolar cell. Remember that light stimulation reduces glutamate release.
- For inhibitory (hyperpolarizing) receptors, a reduction in glutamate release in response to illumination produces depolarization of the bipolar cell.
- For excitatory (depolarizing) receptors, a reduction in glutamate release will hyperpolarize the bipolar cell.

All bipolar cells excite ganglion cells.

The receptive field of a ganglion cell is the region of retina which, when stimulated, affects the firing of the ganglion cell. The size and properties of the receptive field of the ganglion cell are determined by the number of photoreceptors to which it is connected via bipolar cells and the type of synaptic connection formed between the photoreceptor and bipolar cells.

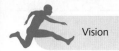
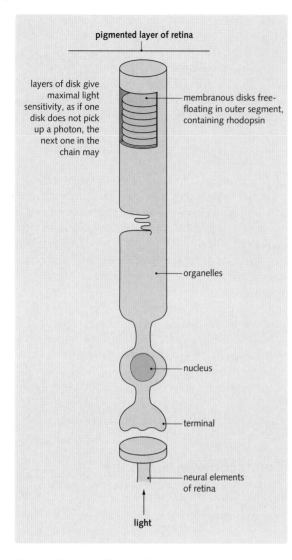

Fig. 8.6 Structure of a rod cell.

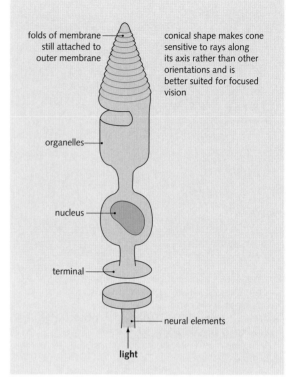

Fig. 8.7 Structure of a cone cell.

- If many receptors converge on a ganglion cell via bipolar cells, its receptive field will be very large, condensing a lot of information into one signal, which is typical of rod connections.
- If a small number of photoreceptors converge on a ganglion cell, its receptive field is smaller and less information is condensed in producing the ganglion output signal, which is typical of cone connections.

The characteristic ganglion cell receptive field is circular, with either an excitatory or inhibitory response elicited from stimulation of the central zone and the opposite response evoked from the surrounding peripheral zone.

Direct receptor–bipolar–ganglion connections produce responses in the central field and connections through horizontal interneurons produce the opposite responses in the peripheral field. These fields are described as having an on-center/off-surround or off-center/on-surround, as shown in Fig. 8.10.

Ganglion cell activity will be greatest when there is a contrast between the center and the surround. If the whole field is illuminated or is in darkness, there is minimal activity because the two antagonistic responses cancel each other. This response pattern helps the visual system to respond to contrast in the visual scene.

There are three types of ganglion cells, which can be distinguished according to their morphology and behavioral properties.

- M cells (magnocellular), which have large cell bodies, thick axons and extensive dendrites, and

Fig. 8.8 Comparison of rods and cones.

	Comparison of rods and cones			
Receptor	**Total number**	**Location**	**Connection to output cells**	**Function**
Rod	120×10^6	peripheral retina, around the fovea	convergent pattern where many rods send information to a few output cells and this compresses information	responding to dim light with low spatial resolution and mediating visual reflexes from stimuli in the peripheral field
Cone	6×10^6	clustered in the fovea	no convergence; each cone projects to one bipolar cell, which projects to one output cell	focused, highly detailed color vision with high spatial resolution

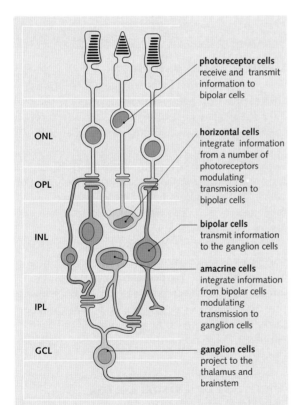

photoreceptor cells receive and transmit information to bipolar cells

horizontal cells integrate information from a number of photoreceptors modulating transmission to bipolar cells

bipolar cells transmit information to the ganglion cells

amacrine cells integrate information from bipolar cells modulating transmission to ganglion cells

ganglion cells project to the thalamus and brainstem

ONL

OPL

INL

IPL

GCL

Fig. 8.9 Processing of visual information in the retinal layers (ONL, outer nuclear layer; OPL, outer plexiform layer; INL, inner nuclear layer; IPL, inner plexiform layer; GCL, ganglion cell layer).

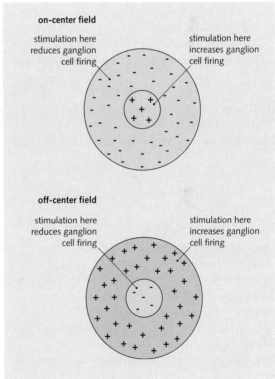

on-center field

stimulation here reduces ganglion cell firing

stimulation here increases ganglion cell firing

off-center field

stimulation here reduces ganglion cell firing

stimulation here increases ganglion cell firing

Fig. 8.10 Receptive fields of ganglion cells.

101

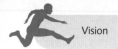
Retinal ganglion cell types					
Ganglion cell	Structure	Receptive field	Response properties	Projection site	Function
X	small cell, small dendritic arbor	small	wavelength specific, slowly adapting	thalamus	signals fine detail and color
Y	large cell, large dendritic arbor	large	rapidly adapting	thalamus, midbrain	signals movement and illumination
W	large cell, large dendritic arbor	large	variable	midbrain	involved in eye movement control

Fig. 8.11 Retinal ganglion cell types.

respond to movement and contrast. These make up some 10% of the population.
- P cells (parvocellular), which have small cell bodies and less extensive dendritic fields. They have smaller receptive fields and respond to color. These make up approximately 80% of the population.
- The remainder have smaller cell bodies than the P cells and thinner axons. They project to the midbrain and are probably involved in reflex adjustment of head and eye position.

Their properties are summarized in Fig. 8.11.

Horizontal integration
Boundaries between light and dark (i.e., edges of objects) are enhanced by the horizontal connections provided by cells in the plexiform layers. The horizontal cells in the outer plexiform layer contact a number of photoreceptors and bipolar cells. Their connections are such that they allow a bipolar cell to be maximally activated when surrounding photoreceptors are not stimulated. Conversely, they inhibit the firing of the bipolar cell when there is photoreceptor activity in the "surround" of its receptive field. This allows edges to be detected.

Synapses formed by amacrine cells in the inner plexiform layer relay signals from rod bipolar cells (which do not directly contact the ganglion cells) to the cone bipolar cells (which do synapse with ganglion cells). This has the function of integrating the responses of rod and cone photoreceptors.

Central visual pathways and the visual cortex

Central visual pathways
The major projection (approximately 90%) from the ganglion cells passes in the optic nerve to the lateral geniculate nucleus of the thalamus, where the axons synapse on cells projecting to the visual cortex.

A smaller projection (approximately 10%) synapses in the midbrain (pretectal area and superior colliculus), controlling visual reflexes and eye movements; there is a small projection from here to higher visual processing areas.

The hemispheres process visual information from only one side of the visual axis (the contralateral), but the optic nerve leaving each eye contains information from both sides of the axis. Some fibers therefore need to cross over the midline so that they project to the contralateral thalamus and this occurs in the optic chiasm anterior to the pituitary stalk, as shown in Fig. 8.12.

Thalamus and visual cortex
The lateral geniculate nucleus
The optic nerve termination in the lateral geniculate nucleus is segregated by eye of origin (thus each lateral geniculate nucleus cell receives monocular information) and by ganglion cell type.

The retinal fibers terminate in six discrete layers—four parvocellular layers (dorsal laminae

Fig. 8.12 Schematic representation of central visual pathways, showing the decussation of nasal fibers in the optic chiasm.

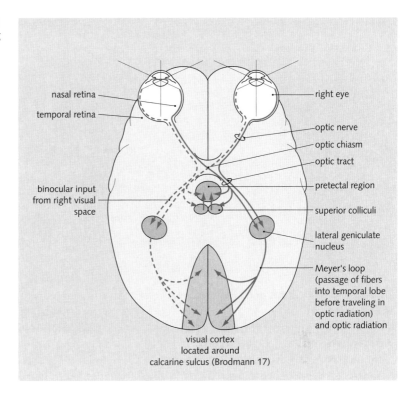

nasal retina

temporal retina

binocular input from right visual space

right eye

optic nerve

optic chiasm

optic tract

pretectal region

superior colliculi

lateral geniculate nucleus

Meyer's loop (passage of fibers into temporal lobe before traveling in optic radiation) and optic radiation

visual cortex located around calcarine sulcus (Brodmann 17)

4–6) and two magnocellular layers (ventral laminae 1 and 2). Each eye transmits to three of the layers with the small-field P ganglion cells projecting to the two parvocellular layers (whose cells are concerned with fine detail), and the large-field M cells to one magnocellular layer (whose cells are concerned with movement). Laminae 1, 4, and 6 receive information from the contralateral eye and 2, 3, and 5 from the ipsilateral eye. This is the first stage of segregation into parallel pathways for form, color, and movement.

The lateral geniculate nucleus has a retinotopic organization, meaning that a given area of the retina will project to only a certain part of the lateral geniculate nucleus. Cells that receive inputs from the same area of the retina are stacked in columns oriented perpendicular to the layers.

Cells in the lateral geniculate nucleus have the same response properties as retinal ganglion cells— small circular fields with center/surround interactions, although the responses to center and surround visual stimuli are much sharper than that seen for retinal ganglion cells.

There are nonretinal inputs to the lateral geniculate nucleus (from the visual cortex and the

pontine reticular formation) that can alter the traffic of information to the visual cortex. This can be used to accentuate information of special interest, which is a mechanism of attention.

The visual cortex

The visual cortex lies along the calcarine sulcus on the medial aspect of the occipital lobe. The lateral geniculate nucleus projects a distorted retinotopic map onto the primary visual area (V1), Brodmann's area 17, so that information from the fovea gains access to a larger volume of cortex (posteriorly) than information from the peripheral retina (anteriorly), as shown in Fig. 8.13.

Similar to other cortical areas, V1 has six layers of cells. Cells in the magnocellular and parvocellular layers in the lateral geniculate nucleus terminate primarily in layer 4 of the V1 cortex. Interestingly, the geniculate projection is double since parvocellular cells project into the lower part of layer 4 whereas the magnocellular cells project into the upper part of layer 4. Other lateral geniculate nucleus cells (interlaminar cells) terminate in layers 2 and 3 on patches of cells termed "blobs" (see below).

103

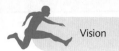
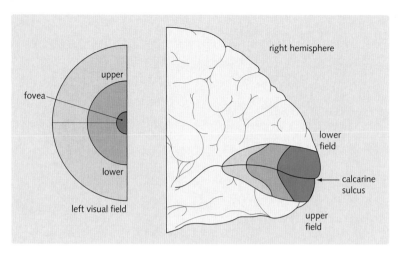

Fig. 8.13 Primary visual cortex—location and representation.

Response of V1 neurons and functional arrangement

Most V1 neurons respond to lines or edges (orientation selectivity), unlike retinal and lateral geniculate nucleus neurons, which have circular receptive fields. Cells that respond to similar line orientations are collected in columns perpendicular to the cortical surface (orientation columns).

Orientation-selective cells can be further classified:

- Simple cells respond to light/dark edges at a specific orientation in a restricted part of the visual field—imagine that they sum the input from a row of adjacent ganglion cells so that the line (light/dark edge or boundary) is formed by the linearly aligned centers of their respective receptive fields.
- Complex cells respond similarly but to activity from a much larger area of the visual field, and maximally to the movement of the edge across the receptive field in a specific direction—imagine that they sum the input from a number of interconnected simple cells.

The orientation columns are grouped together into units that are capable of responding to all orientations of lines in the same part of the visual field in each eye. These units are called hypercolumns, as shown in Fig. 8.14.

Within the hypercolumn, the orientation columns are arranged so that the inputs from the left and right eyes are kept separate, forming so-called ocular dominance columns. This enables higher processing areas to compare the information from both eyes to create depth perception.

Within the hypercolumns, there are regions between groups of orientation columns, called "blob" regions. These are made up of groups of cells responding to color contrast, with the center/surround interaction response pattern to a primary color (center) and its complementary color (surround).

Progression of visual processing

The visual scene that we "see" is built up from different processing circuits in the visual cortex. The latter circuits are formed by pathways coursing through separate areas of the visual cortex each of which contain a retinotopic map. This allows representation of different types of activity in the visual field.

- V2 has an unknown function, but possibly acts as a processing and relay station for higher visual areas.
- V3 may have a role in depth perception and visual acuity.
- V4 has a role in color perception.
- V5 is concerned with motion detection.
- Inferotemporal areas have complex cells that respond to particular stimuli such as faces.

The basis for these theoretical functional areas is the study of individuals with various brain lesions, and of monkeys in which targeted experimental lesions have been made. It was through these kinds of experiment that the concept of parallel pathways came about.

Fig. 8.14 Organization of inputs and outputs in the striate cortex. Diagram shows ocular dominance columns, blob regions, and orientation selectivity (LGN, lateral geniculate nucleus).

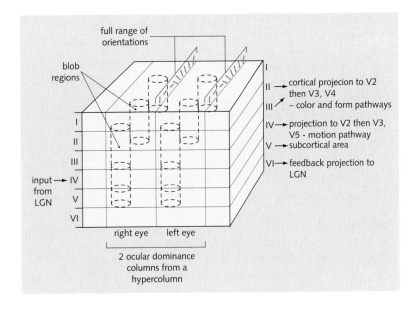

Fig. 8.15 The three parallel visual pathways.

The three visual pathways				
Basic function	Ganglion cell	Visual cortical regions in pathway	Responses of cells	Perceptual role
Motion	Y	V1, V2, V3, V5, then to parietal lobe	rapid responses for moving stimuli, no sensitivity to color	detection of motion and arrangement of objects
From	X	V1, V2, V4, then to parietal lobe and temporal lobe	slowly adapting, some color sensitivity, sensitive to orientation of edges	detection of shape of stationary objects
Colour	X	V1, V2, V4, then to temporal lobe	color-sensitive	detection of color

There are three pathways processing color, motion, and form. The major differences between them are summarized in Fig. 8.15. The circuit that identifies form, the parvocellular or X-cell pathway, is thought to involve more ventral occipitotemporal cortical regions while the circuit involved with motion, the magnocellular or Y-cell pathway, involves more dorsal occipitoparietal cortical areas. The blob system processes color and may be a subset of the parvocellular pathway.

Attention and perception

Attention

The process of attention is the selection of a focus from sensory information in order to process it further. A certain amount of processing of all information has to occur before attentional mechanisms select the appropriate information.

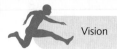

Attending to a part of the environment involves visual and motor mechanisms to orient the body in space, allowing us to scan the visual field or interact with the environment in motor tasks.

The factors that determine where attention is directed are novelty (brightness, color, and change in orientation) and relevance to current tasks.

- The preattentive process is a rapid scanning of a scene to detect objects/gross form.
- The attentive process focuses on specific features of a part of the scene.

Perception

The process of perception involves representing the contents of the environment and then making sense of the representation (e.g., by organizing visual information into objects and background, and then identifying the objects).

Representation of the environment in the visual cortex is achieved by the retinotopic maps. Higher centers know that, if a certain population of V1 neurons are firing, then specific boundaries are present in a specific part of the visual field.

The segregation of visual information into objects and background relies upon certain features of the visual scene. Objects are selected using the following list of principles:

- Common shape, color, or texture.
- Continuity.
- Proximity.
- Common size.
- Closure.
- Depth is extrapolated from a combination of monocular information concerning size, texture, perspective, overlap, movement parallax, and binocular information involving the difference between the view from the eyes and how the eyes move to focus on the same part of space.

The identification of objects, once selected from the environment, relies upon comparison with memories of objects. This occurs in the visual association cortex at the occipitotemporal junction.

Eye movements

Eye movements are important in attentional mechanisms as they direct the fovea toward points of interest in the visual scene quickly and accurately. There are five types of eye movement,

two of which stabilize the eye when the head moves:

- Vestibulo-ocular—uses vestibular input to hold the retinal image stable during brief or rapid head rotation. For horizontal movements, lateral rectus motor neurons (VI nucleus) are influenced by vestibular nuclei cells, medial rectus motor neurons (III nucleus) are driven by interneurons in the contralateral abducens nucleus.
- Optokinetic—uses visual input to hold the retinal image stable during sustained or slow head rotation. The underlying pathway comprises a retinal projection via the tectum to the vestibular nucleus and a cortical component from primary visual cortex.

The other three eye movements keep the fovea on a visual target:

- Saccade—brings new objects of interest onto the fovea. They are very fast and occur every 300 ms. The pattern of saccadic eye movements is guided by current cognitive tasks, as shown by recordings of eye movements when pictures are scanned for details. Horizontal saccadic movements are generated in the pontine reticular formation, and vertical movements are controlled in the midbrain, under influence from a circuit involving the frontal eye fields (in the frontal lobes), the pulvinar nucleus of the thalamus, and the superior colliculus.
- Smooth pursuit—holds the image of a moving target on the fovea. This type of movement is controlled by visual and frontal cortical areas, relaying information to the vestibulocerebellum.
- Vergence—adjusts the eyes for differing image distances. This movement is controlled by midbrain neurons near the oculomotor nucleus. Convergence/divergence of the eyes is induced by blur, and is important in accommodation.

Smooth pursuit movements and saccadic eye movements can alternate (e.g., when looking out of a train window) and this combination of movements is termed optokinetic nystagmus.

Strategies in visual processing

There are two strategies employed by the visual system to comprehend the visual environment:

- Bottom-up processing occurs when a visual scene is analyzed purely in terms of the incoming visual information, without searching visual memory for

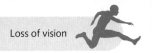

similar scenes that might help with interpreting the scene.

- Top-down processing occurs when visual memory influences the way in which the current visual scene is processed, so that some understanding can be made of the way in which objects are distinguished from their background.

Disorders of attention and perception

In the condition of neglect, patients fail to direct their attention to one half (side) of the visual scene, typically the side of space contralateral to a parietal lobe lesion. The patient will entirely ignore one side of the visual axis (e.g., eating only half the food on a plate) or describe only one half of a visual scene (when actually observing it and when recollecting it).

In the condition of agnosia, patients cannot recognize objects from visual examination, although they can fully describe the physical features of the object (and recognize it from tactile information). Here, there is a failure of the higher processes of perception that integrate all the visual information about an object and compare it with visual memory.

These conditions differ in important respects:
- In agnosia, there is a failure of recognition of an object wherever it is in the visual field.
- In neglect, there is a failure to attend to one half of space, no matter what objects are included.

Loss of vision

Glaucoma

There are two types of glaucoma, which are both characterized by fundoscopic changes, visual field loss, and elevated intraocular pressure. Acute, closed-angle glaucoma is a sight-threatening emergency, whereas primary open-angle glaucoma runs a more chronic and insidious course.

Acute closed-angle glaucoma

This presents as a painful red eye, and may be associated with vomiting. Blurred vision and the appearance of light objects having a "halo" are common in the evenings (when the pupil is dilated). The cause of the rise in intraocular pressure is shown in Fig. 8.16.

Treatment aims to lower the pressure within the eyeball—first medically (e.g., with a pupil constrictor such as pilocarpine), then the flow of aqueous humor

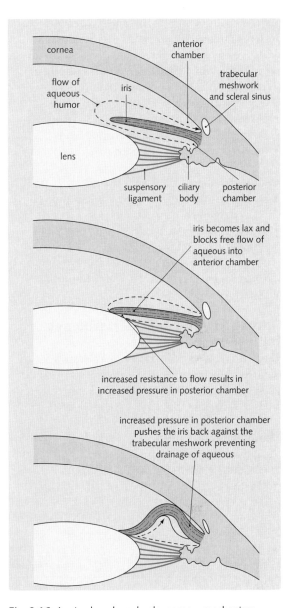

Fig. 8.16 Acute closed-angle glaucoma—mechanism.

from the posterior to the anterior chamber should be restored surgically or with a laser. The other eye should be treated prophylactically.

Primary open-angle glaucoma

This condition is more common than closed-angle glaucoma. The intraocular pressure rises slowly due to a blockage that prevents aqueous humor from entering the trabecular meshwork and canal of Schlemm. As aqueous humor accumulates, intraocular pressure rises and the blood supply to the

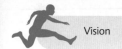

retina is compromised. Symptoms may not be present until severe damage has occurred, and therefore routine screening should be a matter of course, especially for high-risk patients (the elderly and those of African-American origin).

Signs may include:

- Visual field loss.
- "Cupping" of the optic disk on fundoscopy.
- Hemorrhages on the optic disk.

Medical treatment includes the use of:

- β-blockers (topical)—reduces the secretion of aqueous humour.
- Parasympathomimetic agents (e.g., pilocarpine drops)—constrict the pupil.

Laser treatment and surgery may ultimately be necessary.

Damage to the central pathways for vision

The patterns of visual loss following central lesions is primarily dependent on the location of the lesion. These are summarized in Fig. 15.11. Three common types of visual loss are:

Monocular visual loss

Causes:

- Amaurosis fugax (optic nerve ischemia).
- Migraine.

- Temporal arteritis leading to optic nerve infarction.
- Optic neuritis (may be due to multiple sclerosis).
- Rare conditions—methanol poisoning, hereditary optic atrophy, neurosyphilis.

Bitemporal hemianopia

Pressure on the central portion of the optic chiasm caused by:

- Pituitary adenoma.
- Other tumors (e.g., meningiomas).
- Carotid artery aneurysms.

Homonymous hemianopia

Caused by:

- Posterior cerebral artery occlusion and infarction of the occipital cortex.
- May exhibit macular (central) sparing.

Lesions affecting the optic radiations and internal capsule may cause variable degrees of visual loss including homonymous visual impairment affecting just one quadrant. The classic example is a tumor or infarct that involves the ventral and lateral fibers of the optic radiation that extend into the temporal lobe (Meyer's loop) and leads to a homonymous superior quadrantal visual field defect.

Other causes of visual loss are summarized in Fig. 8.17.

Some causes of visual loss	
Acute	**Chronic**
Retinal detachment	Refractive error
Acute closed-angle glaucoma	Cataracts
Retinal artery occlusion (if temporary known as amaurosis fugax)	Corneal disease and edema
Optic neuritis	Primary open-angle glaucoma
Stroke affecting central visual pathways	Age-related macular degeneration
Migraine	Diabetic retinopathy
	Hereditary retinal disease
	Compression of central visual pathways, e.g., tumor
	Drugs: alcohol, methanol, chloroquine

Fig. 8.17 Causes of visual loss.

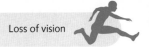

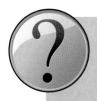

- Describe the functions of the different structures of the eye. What gives it its structural and nutritional support, transparency, and refractive properties?
- What are the structural and functional differences between rods and cones?
- Describe the process of phototransduction.
- How do the retinal cells segregate color information?
- Discuss the visual pathway between the retina and the visual cortex. Why is this organization advantageous?
- Discuss the functional arrangement of the primary visual cortex.
- What is the difference between attention and perception?
- Discuss the role of eye movements in attention.
- Discuss the difference between closed- and open-angle glaucoma. Which should you immediately consider to be an emergency?

9. Hearing

In this chapter, you will learn about:
- The anatomy of the ear.
- How sound waves are transduced into neural signals.
- The central pathways of hearing.
- Special speech areas.
- Deafness and its causes.

The ear and conduction of sound

Sound waves are variations in pressure (i.e., alternating increased and decreased pressure) transmitted through the air.

Sound is principally defined in terms of its amplitude (loudness) and frequency (pitch).

- Amplitude is measured on a logarithmic scale—the decibel (dB)—as there is such a wide variation in the sound intensities the human ear can detect. For human hearing, $dB = 20 \times \log_{10}(P/P_o)$, where P = sound pressure; P_o = the average auditory threshold for frequencies from 1000 to 3000 Hz (20 mpascals or 0.002 dynes/cm^2). Thus, a 20 dB change is equal to a tenfold increase (+20 dB) or decrease (−20 dB) in loudness. Sound pressures greater than 100 dB may damage the cochlea.
- Frequency is measured on a linear scale (cycles/sec or hertz, Hz). Normal hearing occurs over the range from 20 Hz to 20 000 Hz.

The auditory system consists of the hearing apparatus (outer ear, middle ear, and inner ear) and a pathway from the inner ear to the brainstem and auditory cortex.

Anatomy of the auditory apparatus

Fig. 9.1 depicts the auditory apparatus.

Outer ear

The pinna and external ear canal form a tube closed at one end by the tympanic membrane. This tube has a resonant frequency of 3 kHz. The threshold for hearing in the frequency range 2.5–4 kHz is therefore decreased by −15 dB (i.e., these frequencies are easier to hear).

Middle ear

Alternating air pressure (the sound wave) makes the tympanic membrane vibrate. The ossicles vibrate along with it.

- The malleus (hammer) which is attached to the tympanic membrane itself.
- The incus (anvil) which provides a bridge across the middle ear.
- The stapes (stirrup) whose base plate sits in the oval window at the entrance to the cochlea.

The surface area of the base plate is much less (1/17th) than that of the tympanic membrane. Together with the mechanical advantage of the lever system of the incus and malleus (at frequencies near 1000 Hz), this amplifies the pressure changes by 1.3 × 17 or 22-fold (+28 dB). This ensures that sound waves are transmitted efficiently from air to the fluid-filled cochlea.

Vibrations of the ossicular chain are dampened when they become extreme. Two muscles perform this function:

- The tensor tympani muscle on the malleus.
- The stapedius muscle on the stapes.

The reflex contraction of these muscles has a delay of 50–100 msec and cannot protect the cochlea from a sudden loud explosion. The reflex suppresses low frequencies more than high frequencies and may explain how we understand speech in a noisy environment.

The eardrum needs the pressure on either side to be equal for maximum efficiency. The middle ear mucosa constantly absorbs air, and therefore the pressure in the middle ear gradually drops below atmospheric pressure. When it is opened (by swallowing or yawning), the Eustachian tube allows the pressure to equilibrate on both sides of the tympanic membrane. Blockage of this tube leads to a relative hearing defect.

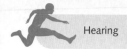

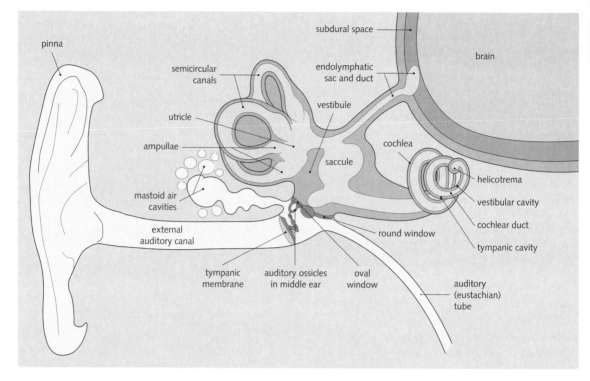

Fig. 9.1 Components and relations of the outer, middle, and inner ear.

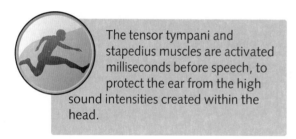

The tensor tympani and stapedius muscles are activated milliseconds before speech, to protect the ear from the high sound intensities created within the head.

Inner ear

The cochlea is a spiral tunnel (with 2.5–3 turns, 32 mm long with a diameter of 2 mm) divided into three compartments running its entire length. The upper compartment (scala vestibuli) and lower compartment (scala tympani) communicate at the apex of the spiral (at the helicotrema). They contain a fluid called perilymph which resembles cerebrospinal fluid. Vibration of the base plate of the stapes causes movement in the perilymph in the scala vestibuli.

The scala media (cochlear duct) lies between the scala vestibuli and the scala tympani, and contains endolymph. Endolymph is a fluid that has a high potassium concentration and therefore a positive potential (80 mV) with respect to the perilymph. The organ of Corti rests on the basilar membrane inside the cochlear duct. The cochlear duct is separated from the scala vestibuli by Reissner's membrane and from the scala tympani by the basilar membrane (Fig. 9.2).

Movement of the perilymph following displacement of the oval window makes the basilar membrane vibrate. This vibration is then transmitted to the hair cells in the organ of Corti, which convert vibrations of their cilia into oscillating changes in their membrane potential. Cranial nerve VIII afferent neurons, whose cell bodies lie in the bony spiral lamina, form synaptic contact with the hair cells and transmit auditory information to the cochlear nuclei in the lateral medulla.

The organ of corti

The ability to detect different frequencies of sound is the function of the basilar membrane and hair cells.

Fig. 9.2 The organ of Corti, lying in the cochlea.

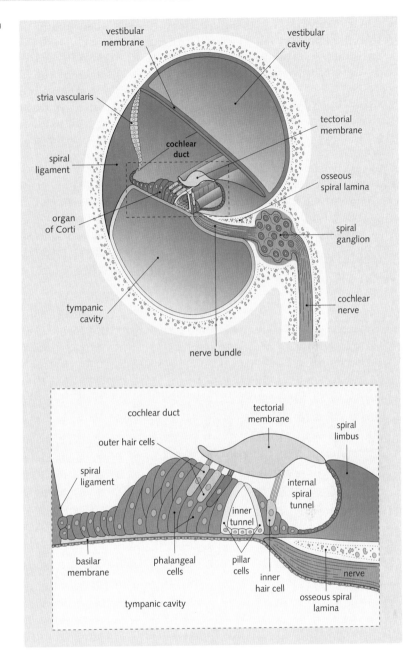

The basilar membrane increases in width as it winds round the cochlea so that its transverse dimension is greater at the apex (500 μm) than at the base (100 μm). This means that lower resonant frequencies are detected at the apex and higher frequencies detected at the base. This is accentuated because the stiffness of the basilar membrane also decreases 100-fold from base to apex.

The electrical and mechanical properties of the hair cells also vary along the basilar membrane. At the base, the hair cells and their stereocilia are short and stiff whereas at the top the hair cells and their stereocilia are more than twice as long and less stiff. The hair cells are thus tuned mechanically and electrically and their ability to generate electrical oscillations matches their mechanical tuning.

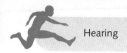
The afferent fibers from the apical part of the cochlea therefore carry low-frequency sound signals, whereas those from the basal part of the cochlea carry high-frequency signals.

Transduction of vibration

The hair cells convert oscillating movements of stereocilia into neuronal signals.

Vibrations of the basilar membrane result in oscillating movement of the hair cells (Fig. 9.3). The stereocilia projecting from the upper surface of the hair cells are fixed at their extracellular end to the immobile tectorial membrane. They sway with the same frequency as the part of the basilar membrane that the hair cells rest upon.

This results in oscillating changes in the physical arrangement of the hair cell membrane and,

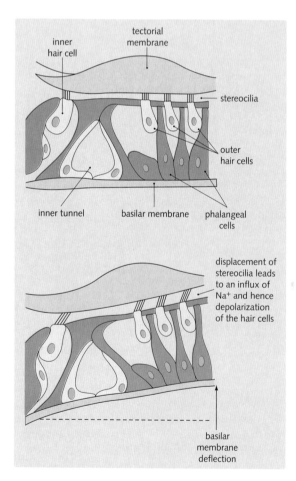

Fig. 9.3 Vibration of the organ of Corti causes bending of hair cell stereocilia, resulting in an oscillating depolarization/hyperpolarization.

consequently, changes in the structure of membrane ion channels. Fluctuations in ion permeability are produced, leading to oscillations of membrane potential with the same frequency as the basilar membrane (note that the maximum firing rate of a nerve fiber has an upper limit of around 500 Hz so that the transduction process is not linear). Interpretation of the signals from the cochlea is due in part to the tonotopic organization of the auditory pathway for frequencies above 4000 Hz and to phase locking of the nerve action potentials for frequencies below 4000 Hz.

Control over sensitivity

Hair cells are arranged in rows on either side of the pillar cells—three rows of outer cells and one row of inner cells. The inner and outer rows have different functions based on the different proportions of output-signalling fibers and input-controlling fibers that contact them.

As a general rule, the bulk of afferent fibers contact the base of the inner cells while efferent fibers (from the superior olivary complex) distribute to either the outer or inner cells. The outer hair cells are contractile and, when activated, may alter their mechanical properties. In this way, they may provide a mechanism for "tuning" the ear to sounds of particular interest. The importance of the outer hair cells can be shown by the fact that excessive exposure to some antibiotics (e.g., gentamicin) can lead to deafness, even though such antibiotics exclusively damage the outer hair cells.

Tonotopic mapping

The spatial separation of frequencies in the cochlea (i.e., each auditory fiber conveys information from a restricted part of the auditory spectrum) leads to frequency selectivity of the cells to which the VIIIth nerve fibers project. Tonotopic mapping occurs as early in the pathway as the projection to the cochlear nuclei. Afferent fibers that arise from the base of the cochlea (high-pitched sounds) penetrate deeply into the nuclei. In contrast, fibers that originate at the apex of the cochlea (low-pitched sounds) terminate in more superficial regions. This is analogous to mapping properties in other sensory systems (e.g., somatotopy).

Sound can be conducted through bone. Thus, after middle ear damage, some hearing is preserved through bone conduction.

The central auditory pathways and the auditory cortex

Central auditory pathways

The pathways are organized so that:

- The tonotopic organization is retained throughout the pathways up to the primary auditory cortex.

- Inputs from both ears interact with each other in the process of sound localization.

Fig. 9.4 shows that VIIIth nerve afferent fibers terminate in the dorsal and ventral cochlear nuclei, at the level of the inferior cerebellar peduncle. From here, there are two main pathways:

- Fibers from the dorsal cochlear nucleus pass in the dorsal acoustic stria, then cross to the opposite

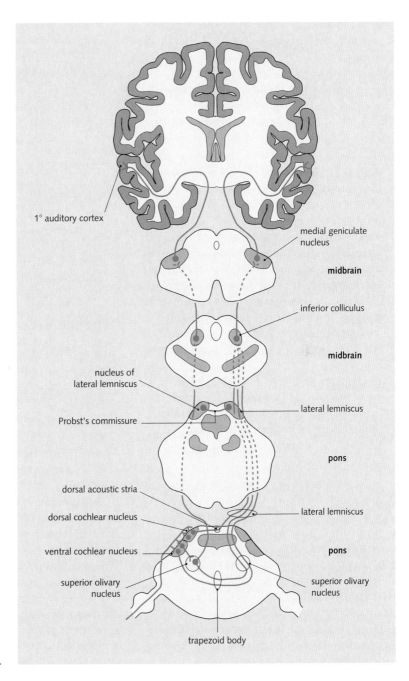

Fig. 9.4 Central auditory pathways.

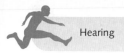

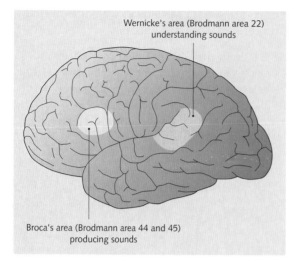

Fig. 9.5 Location of Broca's and Wernicke's areas in the dominant hemisphere.

side to join the lateral lemniscus and terminate in the contralateral inferior colliculus.

- Most fibers from the ventral cochlear nucleus pass ventrally and cross to the opposite side in the trapezoid body. Some fibers project to the superior olivary complex of either side. Others continue rostrally in the lateral lemniscus to the contralateral inferior colliculus. The medial part of the superior olive receives information from both ears and this forms the basis for sound localization. Fibers from the superior olive project bilaterally to the inferior colliculi via the lateral lemnisci.
- Fibers from the inferior colliculus project, ipsilaterally, to the medial geniculate nucleus of the thalamus and, from there, to the ipsilateral primary auditory cortex, on the superomedial aspect of the temporal lobe.

Damage to one side of the central auditory pathway at any level rostral to the cochlear nucleus will not result in deafness in either ear but will result in the inability to accurately localize sound. The absence of deafness is due to the bilateral projections to the auditory cortex, both directly and by communication between pathways.

Auditory cortex

The auditory cortex (Heschel's gyrus, areas 41 and 42) is functionally organized into tonotopic maps that yield the frequency range for normal hearing, with low frequencies represented rostrally and

laterally and high frequencies caudally and medially. This gives rise to isofrequency bands of cells running mediolaterally across the primary auditory cortex.

Cells responding to input from both ears to varying degrees are arranged into columns. Within a column, the cells have a similar frequency response and the same binaural response properties. There are two types of columns, which alternate across the cortex:

- Suppression columns, where cells respond more strongly to input from one ear and are inhibited by input from the other ear. These columns may be involved in sound localization.
- Summation columns, where cells respond to stimulation of both ears, although the input from the contralateral ear is typically greater.

The cortex uses differences in sound intensity and time of arrival at each ear to localize sounds, and the function of each hemisphere is to localize sound from the contralateral side of space.

- From 200 Hz to 2000 Hz, the process involves the delay between a sound reaching one ear and then the other (interaural delay).
- From 2000 Hz to 20 000 Hz, it involves the difference in sound intensity perceived in each ear (interaural intensity differences).

Speech processing

In most individuals, one hemisphere carries out language processing and is called the dominant hemisphere, usually being the left hemisphere for both right-handed and left-handed people.

Wernicke's area in the temporal lobe on the dominant side is an auditory association area that integrates sound information so that meaningful speech can be recognized and comprehended. It codes sounds into phonemes, which are the most basic sound units of spoken language.

Broca's area in the frontal lobe on the dominant side processes the motor programs that are sent to the vocal muscles and produce speech. It matches up a desired phoneme with the motor commands to produce that phoneme.

In speech production, connections between Wernicke's area and Broca's area ensure that the sounds that we wish to make are actually made.

Speech processing also involves other areas, in the frontal, parietal temporal, and occipital lobes (Fig. 9.5).

Fig. 10.3 Influences on the efferent fibers from the olfactory bulb.

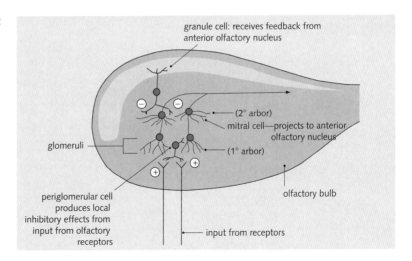

granule cell: receives feedback from anterior olfactory nucleus

(2° arbor)

mitral cell—projects to anterior olfactory nucleus

glomeruli

(1° arbor)

periglomerular cell produces local inhibitory effects from input from olfactory receptors

olfactory bulb

input from receptors

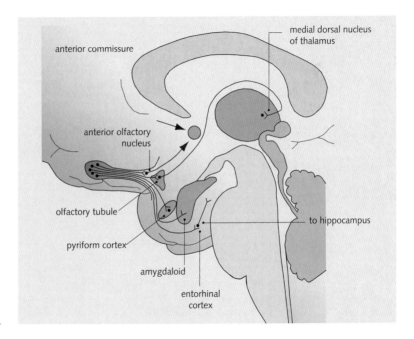

medial dorsal nucleus of thalamus

anterior commissure

anterior olfactory nucleus

olfactory tubule

pyriform cortex

amygdaloid

entorhinal cortex

to hippocampus

Fig. 10.4 Central pathway of smell.

- The entorhinal cortex (parahippocampal gyrus), which projects to the hippocampus (Fig. 10.4).

Central pathways of taste

The taste pathway does not cross the midline and so the hemispheres receive ipsilateral gustatory information.

Taste receptors synapse on afferent neurons of cranial nerve VII, IX, or X, depending on the receptor location. Taste signals from the anterior two-thirds of the tongue are transmitted in the chorda tympani and reach the VIIth cranial nerve. Taste from the posterior one-third of the tongue is transmitted via the IXth nerve. The Xth nerve only sends information from the superior portion of the pharynx. The afferent fibers pass into the medulla where they synapse in the rostral part of the nucleus of the solitary tract, called the gustatory nucleus.

The gustatory nucleus projects to the ipsilateral thalamus (ventroposterior medial nucleus) and from the thalamus there are projections to the sensory cortex and the insula (Fig. 10.5).

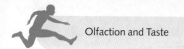

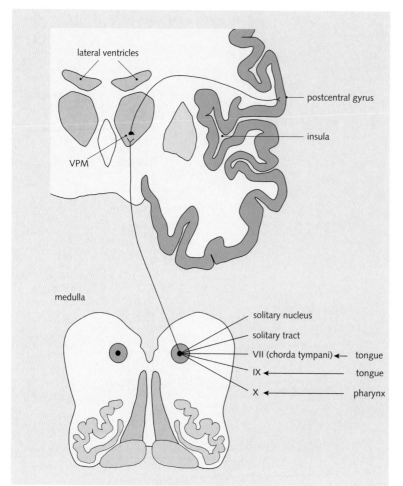

Fig. 10.5 Central pathway of taste (VPM, ventral posterior medial nucleus).

lateral ventricles

postcentral gyrus

insula

VPM

medulla

solitary nucleus

solitary tract

VII (chorda tympani) ← tongue

IX ← tongue

X ← pharynx

There is also be taste input to the hypothalamus and amygdala. Patients with temporal lobe epilepsy often experience gustatory "auras" immediately prior to a seizure.

- Explain briefly the process of olfactory transduction.
- Describe the different taste receptors and their location on the tongue.
- Outline the central pathways of smell. Where are fibers most vulnerable to injury?
- What cranial nerves are involved in the sense of taste?

11. Basic Pathology

In this chapter, you will learn about:
- Cerebral edema, herniation syndromes, and hydrocephalus.
- Congenital diseases of the central nervous system.
- Trauma to the central nervous system.
- Cerebrovascular disease and stroke.
- Central nervous system infections.
- Demyelinating disorders.
- Degenerative disorders.
- Metabolic disorders.
- Brain tumors.
- Epilepsy.

Common pathological features of the central nervous system

Introduction
The bones of the cranium fuse in the first two years of life, making the skull like a rigid box, with a fixed volume.

Intracranial pressure is determined by the volume of the three contents of the skull—brain, cerebrospinal fluid, and blood. None of these three contents is compressible or expandable; therefore, for the intracranial pressure to remain stable, a change in the volume of any of them must be accompanied by an equal and opposite change in the other two. This compensatory mechanism has a limited capacity in terms of speed and magnitude, and its failure results in an increase or decrease in the intracranial pressure (Fig. 11.1).

Cerebral edema
The skull contains approximately 900–1200 mL of intracellular and 100–150 mL of extracellular fluid. An increase in the volume of either of these two components results in cerebral edema.

The pathogenesis of cerebral edema can be divided into three types—vasogenic edema, cytotoxic edema, and interstitial edema. These types of edema usually coexist to variable degrees, depending on the primary pathology.

Vasogenic edema is usually responsive to treatment with corticosteroids, osmotic diuretics, and hyperventilation, whereas cytotoxic edema is often resistant to these therapies. Ultimately, successful treatment relies on identifying and treating the underlying cause.

Vasogenic edema
This is an inflammatory intercellular edema that results from the increased permeability of the capillary endothelial cells. It is caused by either defects in the tight endothelial cell junctions or increased active transport, allowing protein-rich plasma to enter the extracellular space.

Such edema develops around tumors, abscesses, and plaques of multiple sclerosis and affects the white matter predominantly. It may also be seen in trauma, infection, and ischemic areas.

Cytotoxic edema
This is an intracellular edema that results from damage in the ATP-dependent sodium pump, leading to the accumulation of sodium, calcium, and water within the cells (neurons and glia). It affects gray and white matter.

Such edema is commonly seen in hypoxic brain damage and dilutional hyponatremia.

Dilutional hyponatremia may be caused by overenthusiastic fluid replacement or syndrome of inappropriate antidiuretic hormone secretion. In rare cases, patients may simply be drinking far too much water. This can be seen with certain psychological problems and with drug abuse (especially "ecstasy").

Interstitial edema
This is an extracellular edema seen particularly in hydrocephalus. It results from the extravasation of the cerebrospinal fluid through the ependymal cells into the extracellular space of the periventricular white matter.

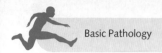

Fig. 11.1 Clinical features of raised and low intracranial pressure.

Clinical features of raised and low Intracranial pressure		
	Causes	Symptoms and signs
raised intracranial pressure	space-occupying masses (e.g., tumor, hematoma, abscess) increase in brain water content (edema) increase in cerebral blood flow volume (e.g., vasodilatation, venous outflow obstruction) increased CSF volume (excessive production, impaired absorption)	early morning headache and vomiting (often without nausea), dizziness, blurred vision, diplopia (usually caused by VI nerve palsy as a false localizing sign), papilledema, focal sensory and motor neurological signs, depressed consciousness, coma, falling pulse rate and rising blood pressure
low Intracranial pressure	decrease in cerebral blood flow volume (e.g., dehydration, blood loss) decrease in CSF volume (e.g., CSF otorrhea and rhinorrhea, lumbar puncture, surgical CSF shunting)	headache and nausea mainly on sitting or standing

> The cerebral circulation autoregulates to maintain blood flow to the brain. It follows the formula: Cerebral perfusion pressure = Mean arterial pressure – Intracranial pressure. Therefore, in conditions such as malignant hypertension, intracranial pressure is increased, and may be very dangerous.

Cerebral herniation

The infoldings of the dura, the falx cerebri (which extends in the midline between the two cerebral hemispheres), and the cerebellar tentorium (the posterior bifurcation of the falx extending laterally over the superior face of the cerebellum with an elongated opening through which the brainstem passes) plus the foramen magnum, divides the brain into semiseparate compartments. When the intracranial volume increases, either due to an increased intracranial pressure or to a space-occupying lesion in any of these compartments, the surrounding brain tissue will be pushed away and forced to herniate into an adjacent compartment, with potentially grave consequences.

Cerebral herniation is divided into four types, as shown in Figs. 11.2 and 11.3.

Hydrocephalus

This is an increase in the cranial cerebrospinal fluid volume. It can be divided into three types:
- Obstructive (noncommunicating) hydrocephalus: caused by a congenital or acquired obstruction in the ventricular cerebrospinal fluid pathway resulting in the accumulation of fluid proximal to the block (Fig. 11.4). It may be relieved surgically by shunting (e.g., ventriculoperitoneal shunt) or by endoscopic ventriculostomy.
- Communicating hydrocephalus: caused by either increased cerebrospinal fluid production or, more commonly, decreased cerebrospinal fluid absorption from the subarachnoid space (Fig. 11.5).
- Normal pressure hydrocephalus: gross ventricular enlargement is seen without cortical atrophy on a computed tomography scan. The pathogenesis is unknown, but may be due to a partial obstruction of cerebrospinal fluid flow from the subarachnoid space. The classical clinical triad is: dementia, gait disturbance, and urinary incontinence.

Symptoms and signs of hydrocephalus are given in Fig. 11.6. Investigations that may confirm hydrocephalus include:

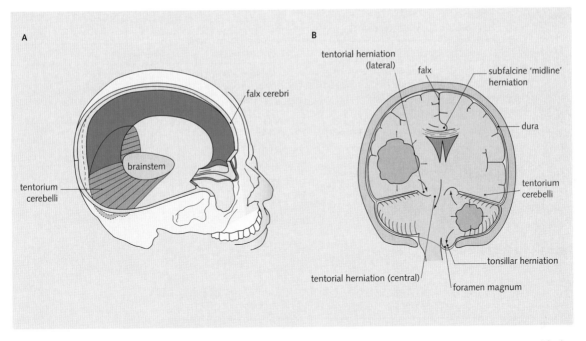

Fig. 11.2 A. The infoldings of the dura mater which compartmentalize the brain tissue. B. Cerebral herniation (modified from *Neurology and Neurosurgery Illustrated* by Dr. Lindsay et al., Churchill Livingstone, 1991).

Types of cerebral herniation		
Clinical type	**Etiology**	**Clinical signs**
type 1: subfalcine herniation	unilateral hemispheric SOL causing that hemisphere to be compressed beneath the falx	frequently seen radiologically, does not usually cause any clinical signs
type 2: lateral tentorial herniation	unilateral hemispheric SOL causing the uncus of the temporal lobe to herniate through the tentorial hiatus; may progress to type 3	ipsilateral third nerve palsy, ipsilateral hemiplegia (contralateral cerebral peduncle compression)
type 3: central tentorial hemiation	midline SOL, very large unilateral hemispheric SOL or bilateral hemispheric diffuse swelling causing a vertical displacement of the diencephalon through the tentorial hiatus; may progress to type 4	impaired upward gaze (pretectum and superior colliculi compression), hemianopia (occipital lobe infarction), hemi/quadriparesis (cerebral peduncle compression), rising blood pressure and bradycardia (aqueduct compression and hydrocephalus), depressed consciousness and respiration (brainstem compression), coma
type 4: tonsillar hemiation	unilateral subtentorial SOL causing herniation of the cerebellar tonsils through the foramen magnum	neck pain, tonic extension of the limbs, cardiac arrhythmia and rising blood pressure, depressed consciousness and respiration, coma

Fig. 11.3 Types of cerebral herniation (SOL, space-occupying lesion).

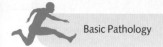

Causes of obstructive hydrocephalus	
Congenital	**Acquired**
aqueduct stenosis	acquired aqueduct stenosis (adhesion following infection or hemorrhage)
Dandy–Walker syndrome	
	intraventricular tumors (colloid cyst, ependymoma) parenchymal tumors (pineal gland, posterior fossa) space-occupying lesion causing tentorial hemiation (see Fig. 14.3)
Amold–Chiari malformation	
vein of Galen aneurysm	
atresia of fourth ventricle foraminae	

Fig. 11.4 Causes of obstructive hydrocephalus.

Causes of communicating hydrocephalus	
Pathogenesis	**Causes**
reduced absorption by arachnoid granulations	infection (especially TB), subarachnoid hemorrhage, trauma, carcinomatous meningitis
excessive CSF production	choroid plexus papilloma
increased CSF viscosity	high protein content

Fig. 11.5 Causes of communicating hydrocephalus.

Symptoms and signs of hydrocephalus		
Age	**Onset**	**Symptoms and signs**
infants and young children	acute	vomiting, depressed consciousness, tense fontanelle, enlarging head, lid retraction and impaired upward gaze ("setting sun sign"), long tract signs
	chronic	mental retardation, failure to thrive, increased skull circumference
adults	acute	signs and symptoms of raised intracranial pressure (see Fig. 14.1), impaired upward gaze
	chronic: communicating hydrocephalus	headache and change in mental status
	normal-pressure hydrocephalus	usually in elderly; dementia, gait disturbance, and urrinary incontinence

Fig. 11.6 Symptoms and signs of hydrocephalus.

- Skull radiography may show changes suggestive of long-standing hydrocephalus (thinning of the skull vault, enlarged pituitary fossa, and erosions of posterior clinoids). This has become second-line due to the advent of computed tomography.
- Head computed tomography/magnetic resonance imaging shows the pattern of ventricular dilatation and excludes the presence of space-occupying lesions.
- Transfontanelle ultrasonography is a useful noninvasive test in neonates.
- Intracranial pressure monitoring (a pressure transducer inserted into the lateral ventricle, brain, or subdural space).

Malformations, developmental disease, and perinatal injury

Neural tube defects

Neural tube defects are caused by varying degrees of failure of fusion of the neural tube and spinal canal. The pathogenesis of the disorders is thought to be due to a mixture of:

- Environmental factors—folic acid (folate) taken at the time of conception and in the first trimester of pregnancy reduces the incidence of neural tube defects. Other factors have not been proven, but it is interesting to note that the incidence in developed countries is much higher than in Asia, despite greater education about the importance of folate supplements.

- Genetic factors—these are complicated in that subsequent children born to a mother with an affected child have a 10-fold increased risk, but monozygotic twins are rarely both affected.

Spina bifida

The lumbosacral site is most common. Spina bifida is caused by local defects in the development and closure of the neural tube and vertebral arches. The main types are shown in Fig. 11.7.

Deficiency of the meninges in these patients predisposes to meningitis. Bladder problems are also common due to a partial cauda equina syndrome.

The spinal cord may be tethered by a fibrous band or tight filum terminale, associated with increasing deficit as the child grows and the cord stretches. Surgery to release the tethered cord may therefore be indicated.

Anencephaly

Anencephaly represents failure of fusion at the cephalic end of the neural tube. Almost no forebrain structures develop, usually with absence of the skull vault. This condition is not compatible with long-term survival.

Arnold–Chiari malformation

Arnold–Chiari malformation is caused by failure of fusion at the craniocervical junction. The brainstem

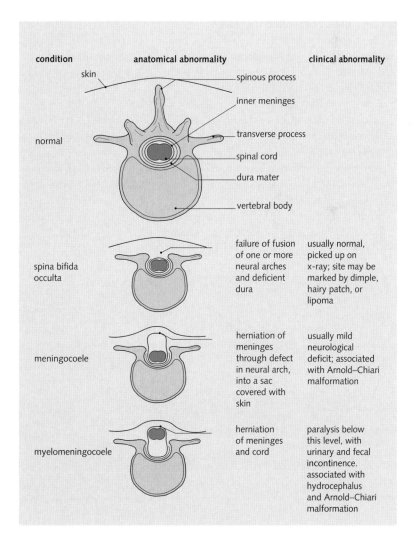

Fig. 11.7 Neural tube defects.

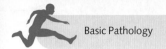

is displaced downward, with the cerebellar tonsils and medulla herniating through the foramen magnum. It is associated with hydrocephalus, especially dilatation of the third and fourth ventricles. Defects may include mental retardation, lower (ocular) cranial nerve palsies, and cerebellar/brainstem signs. Complications include syringomyelia.

Prenatal diagnosis of neural tube defects

Open spina bifida and anencephaly are detectable prenatally by a raised alpha-fetoprotein (AFP). The top 3% of maternal serum AFP levels will include most neural tube defects (as well as many normal fetuses and most twin pregnancies). One in ten pregnant women with a high serum AFP level will have an abnormal baby. Confirmation is with ultrasonography and amniocentesis.

Other congenital diseases

Some other congenital diseases are listed below.

- Microcephaly—which can be developmental or caused by intrauterine infection (e.g., with maternal chickenpox in pregnancy).
- Arteriovenous malformations—these also may be associated with epilepsy or subarachnoid hemorrhage.
- Syringomyelia—a fluid-filled cavity within the cord, sometimes extending to the brainstem (syringobulbia), probably due to many different causes. It is not usually symptomatic until adulthood when it expands, sometimes provoked by a sudden increase in intracranial pressure (e.g.,

a fit of coughing). This is rare, but anatomically interesting. The symptoms of syringomyelia are shown in Fig. 11.8.

- Diastematomyelia—the spinal cord is split in two, sometimes with a bony spur. It presents as a slowly progressive cord syndrome.

 Patients who have had a spinal cord injury are at increased risk of developing syringomyelia many years after the initial injury.

Cerebral palsy

Cerebral palsy is a heterogeneous group of childhood disorders in which injury to the brain early in life results in a nonprogressive neurological disorder of movement and tone (Fig. 11.9). Birth trauma, although the most widely known cause, actually only accounts for approximately 10% of cases. Spastic diplegia is the most common presentation, sometimes with ataxia, hemiplegia, tetraplegia, and dyskinetic syndrome. Other modalities may also be affected, and there may be associated learning difficulties (although intelligence is preserved in up to 70% of patients), visual problems, and epilepsy (30%). Prevalence is approximately two per 1000 live births.

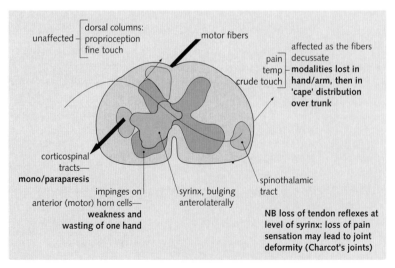

Fig. 11.8 Diagrammatic representation of the cervical cord to explain the symptoms of syringomyelia. Sensory loss is described as dissociated, because pain and temperature sensations are affected, but not joint position and vibration senses. If the cavity extends to the brainstem (syringobulbia), dysarthria, dysphagia, tongue wasting, ataxia, and nystagmus may occur.

Prenatal, perinatal, and postnatal causes of cerebral palsy	
Type	**Cause**
prenatal	intrauterine infection (especially TORCH) difficulties in pregnancy, e.g., preeclampsia, intracranial hemorrhage
perinatal	asphyxia kernicterus
postnatal	infection respiratory distress syndrome

Fig. 11.9 Prenatal, perinatal, and postnatal causes of cerebral palsy.

- Linear fractures.
- Depressed fractures—inner table is depressed by at least the thickness of the skull. The overlying scalp is either intact (simple depressed fractures) or lacerated (compound fractures).

> Basal skull fractures may not be immediately obvious. Signs include bilateral "black eyes," bruising over the mastoid process (Battle's sign), and subconjunctival hemorrhage with no clear posterior margin (indicating blood tracking forward). Avoid nasogasric tubes and nasal airways in these patients.

Trauma of the central nervous system

Epidemiology

Approximately 300 per 100 000 of the population require hospital admission annually for head injuries, with an annual death incidence of nine per 100 000. Approximately one-half of those admitted are under the age of 20 years. The principal causes include motor vehicle accidents, falls, assaults, and industrial, domestic, and sports injuries. Alcohol is frequently involved. Although traffic accidents are the cause of head injury in only 25% of all cases, they contribute to 60% of total fatalities.

Mechanisms

Trauma resulting in brain and spinal cord injuries is of three types:
- Penetrating injuries (e.g., high-velocity missile injuries, gunshot wounds).
- Crush injuries (e.g., industrial injuries).
- Acceleration/deceleration injuries (e.g., motor vehicle accidents).

Brain damage is a result of contusion and laceration of the cerebral cortex, often involving the frontal and temporal lobes. Deceleration injuries also cause diffuse white matter axonal damage.

Skull fractures

Fractures affecting the vault or the base of the skull are an indication that a significant head injury has occurred. They are of two types:

When suspected, a skull radiograph and/or a computed tomagraphy scan should be obtained to confirm the diagnosis.

Complications of skull fractures are:
- Extradural hematoma—often caused by linear fractures crossing the middle meningeal groove and causing the rupture of the middle meningeal artery. This may be indicated by a "lucid interval" after the injury, with a subsequently decreasing conscious level.
- Cerebrospinal fluid rhinorrhea (cerebrospinal fluid leak from the nose)—caused by skull base fractures tearing the dura in the floor of the anterior fossa and the nasal mucosa. This might occasionally be accompanied by pneumatoceles and fluid (visible on radiographs), particularly in the sphenoidal sinuses.
- Cerebrospinal fluid otorrhea (cerebrospinal fluid leak from the ear) caused by fractures of the petrous temporal bone.
- Infection—particularly with compound fractures and persistent cerebrospinal fluid fistulae (cerebrospinal fluid rhinorrhea and otorrhea), in which case prophylactic antibiotic cover is needed.
- Post-traumatic epilepsy—particularly with compound fractures and dural tears causing cortical scarring.

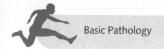

Parenchymal damage

Primary effect

Loss of consciousness is the hallmark of impact brain damage. This might or might not be associated with structural cerebral damage.

Concussion

This term is often used to describe minor head injuries causing temporary loss of consciousness without macroscopic structural cerebral damage. However, microscopic neuronal damage often occurs. The effect of repeated minor head injury is cumulative (e.g., the "punch-drunk syndrome" in boxers).

Contusion/laceration

The skull and the different parts of the brain have different resistances to the movement induced by the accelerating force. When the head is hit by a moving object (or the moving head hits a static object), the brain is accelerated within the skull, and local brain contusion and laceration (coup) occur. This is particularly severe on the undersurface of the frontal and temporal lobes as the brain hits the sphenoidal wing, the petrous temporal bones, and the other noncompliant dural structures. It is usually accompanied by a similar brain injury (contrecoup) at the side directly opposite the local trauma.

Diffuse axonal injury

The combination of linear and rotational acceleration of the brain and the differences in compliance between the white and the gray matter result in tearing of fibers and diffuse axonal injury. This can be identified pathologically by the presence of "axon retraction balls" and microglial clusters, the number of which depends on the duration of survival and the severity of the head injury.

Secondary effect

Impact brain damage is unavoidable; however, head injury induces other delayed pathological processes, which may be preventable and are potentially treatable. The presenting symptoms of these complications depend on the severity of the initial head injury, but they should be suspected if further deterioration in the level of consciousness occurs or new focal neurological signs develop. Note that hemorrhage is a cause of raised intracranial pressure, and may therefore compromise cerebral perfusion. Intracranial pressure monitoring may be indicated.

Intracerebral hemorrhage

Intracerebral hemorrhage arises if arteries or veins crossing the brain tissue are torn. It occurs commonly in the frontal and temporal lobes and is often associated with overlying subdural hemorrhage. In severe head injuries, intracerebral hematoma mixed with necrotic brain tissue might rupture into the dural border (subdural) space, giving a "burst lobe" appearance.

Acute dural border (subdural) hemorrhage

This is a venous hemorrhage caused by tearing of the superficial veins. It is often associated with damage to the surface of the cerebral hemisphere. Pure dural border hemorrhage with no underlying cortical damage can also occur due to the rupture of the veins bridging from the cortical surface to the venous sinuses.

Extradural hemorrhage

This is an arterial hemorrhage caused by skull fractures tearing the middle meningeal vessels. It usually occurs in the temporal and temporoparietal regions. Such a hemorrhage can occasionally be caused by ruptured venous sinuses.

Subarachnoid hemorrhage

Traumatic subarachnoid hemorrhage occurs in most moderate to severe head injuries. Headache, restlessness, and confusion are the most prominent clinical features. It is often difficult to differentiate between traumatic subarachnoid hemorrhage and aneurysmal subarachnoid hemorrhage complicated by depressed consciousness and subsequent head injury.

Cerebral swelling

Cerebral swelling is a common delayed complication of severe head injuries. It may or may not be associated with an intracranial hematoma. The exact mechanism is unknown, but it is often associated with early vasodilatation or an increase in the extracellular or intracellular fluid volume.

Other complications

Other complications are:
- Cerebral ischemia caused by hypoxia, impaired cerebral perfusion, or delayed vasospasm.
- Tentorial and tonsillar herniation caused by raised intracranial pressure.
- Infection presenting as meningitis or brain abscess in association with compound skull fractures.

Chronic dural border (subdura) hematoma
Chronic subdural hematoma presents a different clinical picture compared with acute subdural hematoma. It occurs typically in middle-aged and elderly people. A history of high alcohol consumption is common, but a history of head injury is absent in approximately one-half of cases. Patients present with headache and fluctuating confusion. This should be considered in someone with a vague history of delirium (acute confusional state) or with rapidly progressing symptoms that suggest dementia.

Management
The majority of head injuries are mild and require no specific treatment. In severe head injuries, the principles of management are:
- Adequate airway and oxygenation should be ensured (ensuring that the cervical spine is protected if there is any chance of neck injury).
- Assessment of associated injuries and treatment of hypovolemia should be initiated.

Secondary complications should be managed as follows:
- Intracranial hematomas should be treated with appropriate neurosurgical procedures.
- Cerebral swelling should be treated with mannitol, steroids, and ventilation (to maintain low arterial carbon dioxide).
- Antibiotic cover might be indicated.

Neurological sequelae of head injuries
Common neurological sequelae of head injuries are:
- Retrograde and post-traumatic amnesia.
- Focal neurological deficits.
- Post-traumatic epilepsy.
- Postconcussion syndrome.

Post-traumatic epilepsy
The factors associated with a high risk of post-traumatic epilepsy are:
- Seizures or focal neurological signs in the first week after the head injury.
- Intracranial hematoma.
- Depressed skull fractures, particularly if the dura is torn.
- Post-traumatic amnesia lasting more than 24 hours.

Injuries to the vertebral column and spinal cord
The annual incidence of injuries to the vertebral column and spinal cord is approximately two per 100 000.

In 50% of cases, spinal trauma involves the cervical spine. Injuries to the vertebral column may occur without evidence of cord or spinal nerve injuries; similarly, damage to the neural elements might present without demonstrable injuries to the bone. Neurological damage may result from any of the following four pathological processes:
- Edema, which occurs early and subsides after a few days.
- Hemorrhage—a degree of hemorrhage into the cord (hematomyelia) is almost a constant feature following major spinal trauma. Hemorrhage into the extradural, dural border, or subarachnoid spaces may also occur and could compress the cord.
- Compression of the cord by fractured or misaligned vertebrae.
- Transection of the cord by elements of the vertebral column.

Clinical features depend on the level of injury and the extent of the lesion. The initial spinal shock (transient suppression of nervous function, including reflexes, below the level of injury) begins to subside after a few weeks, and is replaced by spastic weakness.

The principles of management of spinal injuries are:
- Immobilization to prevent further neural damage.
- Preservation of skin integrity (pressure areas).
- Preservation of bladder and bowel function.
- Management of complications (respiratory, cardiovascular, gastrointestinal).
- Long-term rehabilitation—preferably in special centers, which are associated with a better outcome.

Cerebrovascular disease

The risk factors for cerebrovascular disease are:
- Hypertension.
- Diabetes.
- Cardiac diseases: cardiac arrhythmias (particularly atrial fibrillation), valvular heart disease,

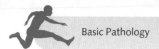

congenital heart disease, and infective endocarditis.
- Obesity, hyperlipidemia, and smoking.
- Alcohol.
- Genetic factors.
- Polycythemia.
- Other factors: male sex, increasing age, previous cerebrovascular disease, illicit drugs, antiphospholipid syndrome, and homocystinuria.

Hypoxia, ischemia, and infarction

There are almost no tissue stores of oxygen or glucose in the brain. When the blood supply fails, the brain ceases to function and cerebral ischemia/infarction occurs.

The normal cerebral blood flow rate is maintained by a number of hemostatic mechanisms at approximately 54 mL/100 g/min, which begins to fail when the mean arterial blood pressure falls below a level of 60–70 mmHg.

Progression from reversible ischemia to infarction depends on the degree and the duration of reduced blood flow. If cerebral blood flow falls below 28 mL/100 g/min, this will result in the development of the morphological changes of infarction. The central necrotic zone of an infarct is surrounded by an "ischemic penumbra"—an area of tissue that is damaged, but remains viable. Restoration of blood flow may therefore give clinical improvement.

Mechanisms of stroke

There are at least four pathological mechanisms underlying atheromatous cerebrovascular disease:
- Atheromatous changes, particularly in the internal carotid artery immediately above the common carotid bifurcation, act as a source of emboli.
- The atheromatous plaque may reach a size sufficient to stenose or occlude an internal carotid or vertebral artery, compromising blood flow.
- Occlusion of small diameter (50–150 mm) penetrating branches of the cerebral arteries by plaques of local atheroma or lipohyalinoid degeneration (seen particularly in hypertension and diabetes) causes small "lacunar" infarcts distal to the occlusion.
- Damage to the walls of small intracranial arteries (lipohyalinoid necrosis) and their subsequent dilatation in hypertensive patients causes small miliary aneurysms (Charcot–Bouchard aneurysms) which may rupture, causing intracerebral bleeding.

Lacunar infarctions and Charcot–Bouchard aneurysms occur most frequently in the following sites:
- The putamen and the internal capsule.
- Central white matter.
- Thalamus.
- Cerebellar hemisphere.
- Pons.

It is often very difficult to differentiate clinically between acute cerebral hemorrhage and infarction, and even pathologically between thrombotic and embolic infarctions.

Definitions
- Transient ischemic attack is a focal neurological deficit of a presumed vascular origin from which a full clinical recovery occurs within 24 hours.
- Reversible ischemic neurological deficit is a focal neurological deficit of a presumed vascular origin from which complete clinical recovery occurs more than 24 hours later.
- Stroke in evolution is a focal neurological deficit of a presumed vascular origin, which progresses over hours or days.
- Completed stroke is a cerebrovascular event with permanent neurological deficit.

Epidemiology

Cerebrovascular disease is a common cause of death after cardiovascular and malignant disease. The majority of strokes are ischemic.

Clinical features
Transient ischemic attack

Transient ischemic attacks are generally of thromboembolic etiology. They should be recognized and managed promptly because they are an indication that a full stroke may be imminent. Carotid territory transient ischemic attacks present with:
- Transient monocular blindness (amaurosis fugax).
- Transient sensory or motor symptoms of the face, arm, or leg.
- Transient aphasia.

Spinal abscess

Spinal abscesses are epidural in two-thirds of cases. One-half of the cases result from hematogenous spread of skin or urinary tract infections, and the remainder from direct spread from vertebral osteomyelitis. *Staphylococcus* is the commonest causative organism, followed by *Escherichia coli* and *Proteus*. Clinical features:

- Severe localized spinal pain.
- Fever.
- Signs of spinal cord compression.

Magnetic resonance imaging is the investigation of choice for spinal imaging.

Spinal abscesses should be treated with immediate surgical decompression and antibiotics.

Chronic meningoencephalitis
Tuberculous meningitis

Tuberculous meningitis is uncommon in developed countries, with an annual incidence of 0.2 per 100 000. It is more common in socially and economically deprived communities.

Clinical features include:

- Prolonged prodromal illness followed by slowly evolving meningeal symptoms.
- Adhesive arachnoiditis causing cranial nerve palsies and hydrocephalus.
- Localized vasculitis and caseation causing focal neurological signs and seizures.

Investigations:

- A head CT should be performed in patients with focal neurological signs or depressed consciousness.
- Cerebrospinal fluid examination shows raised lymphocyte count, high protein, and low glucose.
- Ziehl–Nielsen staining occasionally reveals the presence of acid-fast bacilli, which will be confirmed by culture.

Treatment:

- A combination of isoniazid, rifampicin, and pyrazinamide.
- Pyridoxine is given to prevent isoniazid-induced neuropathy.
- Corticosteroids may also be given initially to reduce the host inflammatory response.

Mortality:

- Mortality is very high, reaching 20–30% in treated patients.
- Many survivors are left disabled.

Neurosyphilis

Treponema pallidum (a spirochete) invades the central nervous system within 3–24 months of the primary infection in 25% of untreated cases. Although the incidence of neurosyphilis has declined, it is important to maintain a high diagnostic suspicion since neurosyphilis may mimic other common neurological disorders.

Clinical features include:

- Asymptomatic meningeal neurosyphilis.
- Meningovascular syphilis—acute hemiplegia and sudden individual cranial nerve palsies.
- Tabes dorsalis—proprioceptive sensory loss, with unsteady, wide-based gait.
- General paralysis (of the insane)—dementia and upper motor neuron paralysis of the limbs.
- Neurosyphilitic gummata (rubbery granulomata) themselves may cause seizures and focal neurology when they are present in brain tissue.

Abnormal pupils (Argyll–Robertson) should be looked for, along with absent knee or ankle jerks and a positive Babinski sign. A consideration of whether the patient is at high risk of being HIV positive should be made, and appropriate precautions taken.

Lyme disease

Lyme disease is a spirochetal infection caused by *Borrelia burgdorferi*, classically after an *Ixodes* tick bite. It presents initially with a characteristic skin rash (erythema chronicum migrans). Fifteen per cent of patients develop neuroborreliosis, which may mimic other common neurological disorders:

- Chronic meningitis.
- Encephalitis.
- Cranial nerve palsies (particularly facial).
- Painful radiculopathy.
- Peripheral neuropathy.
- Mononeuritis multiplex.

Treatment is with a cephalosporin with good central nervous system penetration (e.g., ceftriaxone)

Viral encephalitis

Viral encephalitis is an acute febrile encephalitic illness that is often associated with a meningeal component. It can be caused by many viruses, including mumps, herpes simplex and zoster, Epstein–Barr, Coxsackie virus and echo viruses. Herpes simplex encephalitis (HSE) is particularly important because it is treatable.

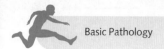

Clinical features:

- Headache, fever, altered consciousness.
- Occasionally, acute psychiatric symptoms (delusions, hallucination), seizures, or focal neurological signs.
- Hemispheric signs (e.g., dysphasia, hemiparesis) are more likely in herpes simplex infection.

Encephalitis is inflammation of the brain parenchyma itself, without involvement of the meninges. In reality, there is generally some meningeal involvement in encephalitis and vice versa.

Investigations:

- A head CT or MRI excludes space-occupying lesions and may show focal abnormalities in the affected lobes (particularly the temporal lobe in HSE).
- Cerebrospinal fluid examination shows a raised lymphocyte count, with slightly raised protein and normal glucose, but may be entirely normal.
- Electroencephalogram (EEG) shows diffuse slow activity (delta waves), with focal periodic complexes (in HSE).
- Blood and cerebrospinal fluid may show rising viral antibody titers.
- Viruses may be identified in the cerebrospinal fluid (culture, polymerase chain reaction).

Treatment:

- Acyclovir is very effective in HSE. It is relatively nontoxic and should be used whenever this diagnosis is suspected.

Prognosis:

- Varies according to the causative virus.
- If untreated, the overall mortality of herpes simplex encephalitis is approximately 70%, which can be reduced to 20% with acyclovir.

Other virus-induced neurological diseases

For clinical purposes, viral illnesses are best considered by the clinical syndrome they produce (Fig. 11.13).

Fungal infections

Fungi are frequently the cause of opportunistic infections in immunocompromised patients, particularly in those with HIV. The most common fungi associated with central nervous system infection are *Cryptococcus*, *Nocardia*, *Candida*, and *Aspergillus*. Fungal infection commonly presents with subacute meningitis complicated by cortical thrombophlebitis and cerebral abscesses. Cerebrospinal fluid examination shows moderate polymorphonuclear leukocytosis, increased protein, and low glucose. The causative fungi can be demonstrated on Gram or Indian-ink staining, or by using special culture techniques.

Treatment is with antifungal agents, but mortality and morbidity are high.

Protozoan infection

Toxoplasma

Toxoplasma gondii is an intracellular protozoan parasite. Humans are occasionally infected through the ingestion of raw uncooked meat or cat feces, or by the transplacental route. Congenital toxoplasmosis, caused by transplacental transmission, presents with hydrocephalus, hepatosplenomegaly, retinochoroiditis, and thrombocytopenia.

Acquired toxoplasmosis occurs in immunocompromised patients (particularly in AIDS), with features of meningoencephalitis, seizures, focal neurological signs, and depressed consciousness. Head CT in acquired toxoplasmosis shows characteristic contrast-enhancing lesions.

Toxoplasma immunoglobulin G antibodies are found in most patients. Brain biopsy is diagnostic. Mortality is very high (70%).

Malaria

Cerebral malaria, causing a hemorrhagic encephalitis, is caused by *Plasmodium falciparum*. The main clinical features consist of fever and malaise, followed 2–3 weeks after initial infection by severe headache, deleirium, seizures, progressive stupor leading to coma and, occasionally, focal neurological signs.

The diagnosis is established by showing malarial parasites in erythrocytes on a thick and thin blood film.

Treatment is with intravenous quinine. Mortality is high (22%).

Other virus-induced neurological diseases		
Virus	**Neurological syndrome**	**Principal symptoms**
Varicella zoster	Shingles	Painful vesicular eruption in dermatomal distribution
Retroviruses HTLV1, HIV	Tropical spastic paraparesis, AIDS	Spastic paraparesis, meningitis, myeolpathy, neuropathy, dementia
Measles	Acute: meningoencephalitis Chronic: subacute sclerosing, panencephalitis (SSPE)	Deteriorating intellect, seizures, pyramidal signs
Rabies	Rabies	Psychiatric symptoms (affective disorders), hydrophobia/aerophobia, hyperreflexia, and spasticity or ascending paralysis mimicking Guillain–Barré syndrome
Papoviruses (JC, SV40)	Progressive multifocal leukodystrophy	Dementia in an immunocompromised patient
Arboviruses	Postencephalitic parkinsonism	Parkinsonism syndrome with dystonic movement disorders
Rubella	Progressive rubella encephalitis	Mental retardation, seizures, optic atrophy, cerbellar and pyramidal signs
Poliovirus	Poliomyelitis	Meningeal irritation, asymmetric paralysis without sensory involvement

Fig. 11.13 Other virus-induced neurological diseases.

Prion diseases

Creutzfeld–Jakob disease (CJD) is thought to be caused by an infectious prion protein, and leads to a spongiform encephalopathy. Inherited CJD is an autosomal dominant trait, but most cases are sporadic. The "new variant" CJD, which has provoked such intense media interest, may have a connection with bovine spongiform encephalopathy in cattle. As yet, there is no indication of how this disease has "jumped" species. Evidence comes from the fact that infected brain tissue from cattle can cause a spongiform encephalopathy when injected into the nervous system of various species, including cats. It is interesting to note that there has been no documented increase in the number of cases of feline spongiform encephalitis. This is despite the fact that cats almost certainly have eaten more contaminated beef than humans.

New variant CJD tends to affect younger patients, and presents initially with psychiatric disturbance and ataxia. Dementia invariably follows, and death occurs within 1–2 years. It is still extremely rare.

Demyelination and degeneration

Demyelination
Multiple sclerosis

Multiple sclerosis (MS) is a chronic disorder in which episodes of inflammatory demyelination affect any part of the central nervous system, producing a variety of symptoms. It has an extremely variable course with a tendency toward progressive disability.

MS cannot be diagnosed until the patient has suffered multiple attacks at different neuroanatomical sites.

Incidence and prevalence

The incidence and the prevalence of MS vary markedly between the different geographical areas

139

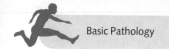

throughout the world and the different population groups.

Etiology

The etiology of MS is unknown, but is likely to involve environmental factors (e.g., a viral infection) in genetically susceptible patients. There also is a human leukocyte antigen association, leading to theories of an autoimmune basis. The pathological hallmarks are scattered demyelinating lesions in the perivenous areas of the white matter of the brain and the spinal cord, referred to as "plaques."

Symptoms and signs

Depending on the anatomical location of the plaques, four main groups of symptoms are recognized:

- Optic nerve: attacks of optic neuritis presenting with blurring of vision associated with periorbital and retro-orbital pain exacerbated by eye movements, reduced visual acuity, central scotoma, afferent pupillary defect, and a pink and swollen optic disk (which becomes pale and atrophic at a later stage).
- Brainstem: diplopia; dysconjugate eye movements, particularly internuclear ophthalmoplegia; limb and gait ataxia, titubation, tremor, dysarthria, and vertigo.
- Spinal cord: sensory symptoms including Lhermitte's phenomenon (electric-shock-like sensation extending down the spine into the limbs on neck flexion); spastic weakness; bladder, bowel, and sexual dysfunction.
- Other clinical features: dementia, euphoria, and emotional lability; facial pain; painful tonic spasms; Uhthoff's phenomenon (transient worsening of symptoms following a hot bath or exercise).

Investigations:

MS is a clinical diagnosis and no test is pathognomonic. Cerebrospinal fluid shows oligoclonal bands in almost all cases. Evoked potentials (visual, auditory, and somatosensory) may be prolonged. Magnetic resonance imaging is abnormal in almost all patients.

Treatment:

Acute relapses are treated with oral or intravenous steroids. Analgesia and baclofen may reduce spasticity. Bladder symptoms may require specialist referral. Interferon-β is effective in reducing relapse rate, but has no proven effect on long-term disease progression. It is not effective in all patients, and is extremely expensive. Therefore, its use should be reviewed regularly.

Prognosis:

The average duration of the illness to death is 25–30 years.

Other demyelinating conditions

Acute disseminated encephalomyelitis may follow many common viral infections, and causes focal brainstem and spinal cord demyelination that resembles MS. The prognosis is variable—from complete recovery to 25% mortality in severe cases.

Central pontine myelinosis is associated with alcoholism and hyponatremia. It presents acutely with pontine and medullary symptoms. It is treated by correcting underlying metabolic abnormalities and with vitamins. Prognosis is poor.

Degenerative diseases
Degenerative diseases in which dementia is prominent (cortical dementia)
Alzheimer's disease

Alzheimer's disease is the most common cause of dementia, accounting for 80% of all cases of dementia in the community. The incidence increases with age; familial cases are occasionally seen. The female : male ratio is 3 : 1.

Clinical features are those of cortical dementia:
- Memory impairment (particularly of recent events), apathy, poor reasoning and judgment.
- Behavioral disturbance (aggression is often prominent).
- Aphasia, apraxia, spatial disorientation.
- Eventually patients become mute, bedfast, and incontinent.

The main pathological changes are:
- Considerable brain atrophy, most evident in the superior and middle temporal gyri.
- Neurofibrillary tangles: intracellular paired helical filaments which are particularly common in hippocampal, amygdaloid, and pyramidal neurons.
- Neuritic plaques: extracellular areas of degenerating neuronal processes surrounding a central core of β-amyloid protein.

- Loss of cholinergic neurons in the medial septal nucleus, the horizontal nucleus, and nucleus of diagonal band.

The cause(s) of Alzheimer's disease is not known, although genetic predisposition is likely to be very important. Risk is increased by three times in first-degree relatives. The high prevalence of Alzheimer's in Down's syndrome suggests that the gene that encodes the β-amyloid precursor, on chromosome 21, is one of the most important candidate genes. A specific isoform of the lipid transport protein, apolipoprotein E, is an independent risk factor for the development of Alzheimer's disease; its gene is located on chromosome 19.

Investigations, which are largely undertaken to exclude other, treatable, causes of dementia, include:

- Imaging (computed tomography, magnetic resonance imaging) which shows brain atrophy, flattening of the gyri, widening of the sulci, and dilatation of the ventricles. This will also help to exclude vascular causes of dementia which can be prevented from progressing.
- B_{12}/folate levels and thyroid function tests.

Pick's disease

Pick's disease is another form of dementia which may be indistinguishable from Alzheimer's until autopsy. Classically, it is dominated by frontal and temporal lobe symptoms. Treatment is the same.

Treatment:

- Maintenance of general health—concurrent illnesses (including affective disorders) may exacerbate symptoms.
- Avoidance of sedative drugs.
- Treatment should be considered using an inhibitor of acetylcholinesterase which may slow cognitive decline in some patients.

Prognosis:

- Most patients die from the complications of immobility within 5–10 years of diagnosis.

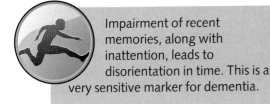

Impairment of recent memories, along with inattention, leads to disorientation in time. This is a very sensitive marker for dementia.

Degenerative diseases in which extrapyramidal features are prominent (subcortical dementia)

Parkinson's disease

The annual incidence is 1 in 5000, with a prevalence of about 1 per 500. Age of onset is generally approximately 50 years onwards, but 8% of patients develop symptoms before the age of 40 years. The cause remains unclear, although genetic (particularly in early-onset Parkinson's) and environmental factors are likely to be important.

The main pathological changes are:

- Loss of the pigmented cells in the substantia nigra which results in severe striatal dopamine deficiency.
- Atypical eosinophilic inclusion bodies, called "Lewy" bodies.

Clinical features:

- Bradykinesia as the cardinal feature. Patients present with slowness of gait, difficulties in writing and using their hands or turning in bed, and reduced facial expression.
- Resting tremor classically of four or five cycles per second.
- Rigidity of lead-pipe or (with superimposed tremor) cogwheeling type.
- Impaired postural control and loss of righting reflexes, causing flexed posture and falls in advanced cases.
- Dementia in approximately 30% of cases.
- Affective disorders are very common—particularly anxiety and depression.

Differential diagnosis:

- Benign essential tremor.
- Depression and motor retardation.
- Drug-induced parkinsonism.
- Other degenerative disorders.
- Progressive supranuclear palsy (Steele–Richardson–Olszewski syndrome)—characterized by more tone in the neck than the limbs and falls early on in the disease.
- Wilson's disease—a disorder of copper metabolism.
- Diffuse Lewy body disease.
- Alzheimer's disease.
- Diffuse cerebrovascular disease with abnormal gait.

Investigations:

- The diagnosis is usually based on the clinical features and response to treatment.

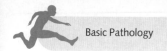

- Imaging, autonomic function tests, and sphincter electromyogram are occasionally needed to exclude other parkinsonian syndromes.

Treatment:
- Anticholinergic and dopaminergic drugs are the main line of treatment. These are discussed in Chapter 5.
- Dopaminergic neuronal implantation is still a research procedure.

Prognosis:
- With treatment, life expectancy is now only slightly worse than that of the general population.

Huntington's disease

Huntington's disease is an autosomal dominantly inherited disorder. The gene is on chromosome 4. The prevalence is approximately 8 per 100 000, and onset is usually in middle age. Pathologically, there is neuronal loss in the striatum associated with deficiency of γ-aminobutyric acid (GABA), acetylcholine, enkephalin, and substance-P.

Onset is insidious, with:
- Chorea (writhing, dance-like movements).
- Affective disorder and personality changes.
- Dementia of subcortical type.

Investigations:
- The clinical diagnosis is usually confirmed with genetic studies.
- Head CT or MRI in advanced cases show atrophy of the caudate nuclei.

Treatment:
- No specific treatment is available. Chorea is treated symptomatically with neuroleptics (e.g., haloperidol).
- Genetic counseling of the affected families is essential.

Prognosis:
- Most patients die from aspiration within 10–20 years of diagnosis.

Hereditary ataxias and related disorders

These heterogeneous disorders present with progressive ataxia as a predominant clinical feature (Fig. 11.14).

Motor neuron disease

The annual incidence of motor neuron disease is approximately 2–3 per 100 000. It usually presents between the ages of 50 and 70 years. Three major types are recognized:

Hereditary ataxias		
hereditary ataxia of known cause	intermittent ataxia	disorder of urea cycle disorders of lactate and pyruvate metabolism (Leigh's disease)
	progressive ataxia	abetalipoproteinuria ataxia telangiectasia xeroderma pigmentosa
	spinal ataxia	Friedreich's ataxia
hereditary ataxia of unknown cause	cerebellar ataxia	pure cerebellar degeneration

Fig. 11.14 Hereditary ataxias.

- Amyotrophic lateral sclerosis: the classical form of motor neuron disease—this is a combination of upper and lower motor neuron limb and cranial nerve weakness.
- Progressive muscular atrophy: a lower motor neuron limb weakness.
- Progressive bulbar palsy: a combination of upper and lower motor neuron cranial nerve weakness.

These syndromes represent a continuum, and patients progress from one syndrome to the other. Sensory symptoms and signs are usually absent. Treatment is aimed at maintaining a reasonable quality of life for as long as possible using a multidisciplinary approach. Prognosis is extremely poor and the survival is approximately 2–3 years.

Spinal muscular atrophy (SMA)

SMA is a group of hereditary conditions characterized by progressive lower motor neuron degeneration. Features include hypotonia, proximal weakness, and wasting. There are four main types:
- Acute infantile SMA (Werdnig–Hoffmann disease)—presents at birth or shortly after, death is by age 3 years.
- Chronic infantile SMA—presents at 6 months, death is by 10 years.
- Juvenile onset SMA (Kugelberg–Welander disease)—presents at approximately 10 years, death is around 35 years.
- Peroneal/scapuloperoneal SMA—adult onset, survival is roughly normal.

Metabolic disorders and toxins

Vitamin deficiencies

Nutritional vitamin deficiencies are rare in developed countries and are usually seen in chronic alcoholics and socially isolated people, including elderly or mentally ill patients. Vitamin deficiency can also result from diseases (malabsorption, autoimmunity) or drugs (isoniazide), and is usually not limited to a single vitamin in isolation. Some common features and causes of vitamin deficiencies are shown in Fig. 11.15.

Vitamin overdose (vitamin A) occasionally results in neurological complications (headache, papilledema).

Toxins
Methanol

Poisoning with methanol causes headache and photophobia and, in severe cases, papilledema, optic atrophy, and blindness. Ethanol infusion (ethanol competes with methanol) and hemodialysis are the mainstays of treatment.

Alcohol

Neurological complications of alcoholism include:

- Acute intoxication. The effect of acute alcohol administration depends on the amount of alcohol consumed and on whether the subject is a naïve or chronic alcohol user. The symptoms range in

Clinical features and common causes of vitamin deficiencies			
Vitamin	**Function**	**Cause**	**Neurological sequelae**
A	essential for normal retinal and epithelial cell function	malnutrition	adults and children: blindness infants: mental retardation and hydrocephalus
B_1 (thiamine)	pyruvate metabolism	malnutrition, alcoholism	Wernicke's encephalopathy, Korsakoff psychosis, neuropathy
B_3 (nicotinic acid)	NAD, NADP coenzyme component	malnutrition	encephalopathy, neuropathy
B_6 (pyridoxine)	cofactor in protein metabolism	malnutrition, isoniazide treatment	neuropathy, seizures (infants)
B_{12} (cobalamine)	purine synthesis	autoimmunity, ileal disease, gastrectomy, malnutrition	dementia, myelopathy (subacute combined degeneration), neuropathy
folic acid	purine synthesis	malabsorption, malnutrition	myelopathy, neuropathy, neural tube defect
D	calcium metabolism	malabsorption, malnutrition, chronic renal failure	myopathy
E	antioxidant	malabsorption	cerebellar ataxia

Fig. 11.15 Clinical features and common causes of vitamin deficiencies.

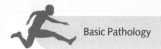

severity from euphoria and mild incoordination to ataxia, dysarthria and confusion, to deep anesthesia and respiratory suppression. Secondary effects of intoxication include head injury, hypoglycemia, and hyponatremia. The possibility of other drugs should be considered.

- Alcohol withdrawal syndrome (tremors, hallucinations, seizures, and delirium tremens). Action tremor usually reaches a peak 24–36 hours after the cessation of drinking, and is promptly aborted by further alcohol intake. Hallucinations may be visual, auditory, or tactile. Seizures occur 24–48 hours after the cessation of drinking. Delirium tremens combines the three previous features and severe autonomic overactivity (dilated pupils, pyrexia, tachycardia, and sweating).
- Nutritional complications (Wernicke–Korsakoff syndrome—caused by thiamine vitamin B_1 deficiency, and neuropathy). Early clinical features are those of ataxia, oculomotor disturbances (oculomotor palsies and nystagmus), and confusion which, if untreated, can progress to coma and death. As the patient's confusion improves following treatment, the amnesic component of the syndrome emerges in which confabulation is a prominent feature. Neuropathy is a symmetrical sensorimotor axonal neuropathy.
- Hepatic complications (acute hepatic encephalopathy and chronic portosystemic encephalopathy).
- Other syndromes: dementia/brain atrophy; alcoholic cerebellar degeneration (characterized by gait and truncal ataxia); alcoholic myopathy (acute painful proximal myopathy); central pontine myelinolysis (acute syndrome of quadriparesis, pseudobulbar palsy occasionally associated with abnormal eye movements and "locked-in" syndrome).

Carbon monoxide poisoning

The high affinity of hemoglobin to carbon monoxide results in severe tissue hypoxia. Acute intoxication leads to acute encephalopathy with visual field defects, papilledema, and retinal hemorrhage. Many patients are left with chronic encephalopathy and parkinsonism. Hyperbaric oxygen may help to prevent this, even hours after exposure.

Heavy metals
Lead

Acute encephalopathy is seen largely in children. Chronic motor neuropathy typically presents with wrist drop.

Mercury

Mercury causes chronic encephalopathy with ataxia, dysarthria, and tremor.

Manganese

Manganese causes chronic encephalopathy and parkinsonism.

Iatrogenic
Drugs

Drug-induced neurological disorders include:
- Encephalopathy (e.g., hypnotics, sedatives, antidepressants in large doses).
- Neuropathy (e.g., isoniazide, vincristine).
- Neuromuscular transmission blockade (e.g., penicillamine).
- Myopathy (e.g., steroids).
- Extrapyramidal syndrome (e.g., antipsychotic medications and antiemetics).
- Psychiatric symptoms (e.g., antiparkinsonian medications).

Neurological complication of opiate abuse:
- Acute intoxication
- Withdrawal syndrome
- Transverse myelitis
- Neuropathy:
  - Acute painful plexopathy
  - Acute mononeuropathies/mononeuritis multiplex
- Myopathy:
  - Rhabdomyolysis
  - Chronic myopathy
- Infection:
  - Cerebral abscess
  - Mycotic aneurysm

Radiotherapy

Neurological complications are related to the total radiation dose and the period over which it is given.

Early features are related to localized edema. Delayed features are related to necrosis, which often simulates tumor recurrence.

Neoplasms of the central nervous system

Primary brain tumors

The annual incidence of primary brain tumors is about 8.2 per 100 000, accounting for about 5% of all neoplasms in the body. However, they make up approximately 50% of all childhood malignancies.

The prevalence of the different tumor types and their anatomical location varies with age:
- Adults: gliomas, metastases, and meningiomas.
  - 80–85% supratentorial compartment.
  - 15–20% infratentorial compartment.
- Children: medulloblastomas and cerebellar astrocytomas.
  - 40% supratentorial compartment.
  - 60% infratentorial compartment.

The clinical features depend on the site of the tumor and the speed of growth, and can be divided into three main categories:
- Features of raised intracranial pressure (headache, vomiting, and papilledema).
- Focal symptoms and signs, the nature of which depends on the anatomical site of the tumor and whether the tumor effect is irritative or destructive.
- False localizing signs due to raised intracranial pressure (e.g., VIth nerve palsy).

Neuroepithelial tumors
Astrocytomas

Astrocytomas are the most common primary tumors of the brain. They can occur at any age, but are most frequent between the ages of 40 and 60 years. Male/female incidence is 2 : 1. Astrocytomas occur with equal incidence throughout the frontal, temporal, and parietal lobes, but are uncommon in the occipital lobe.

There are four pathological grades (Kernohan I–IV):
- Low-grade astrocytoma (grades I and II)—commonly seen in children/young adults.
- Malignant astrocytoma (grade III).
- Glioblastoma multiformis (grade IV).

Sadly, malignant astrocytomas are far more common than benign ones.

Oligodendroglioma

Oligodendroglioma is a slow-growing tumor with low malignancy grade. It affects a younger age-group (30–50 years) and is most common in the frontal lobe. Imaging reveals a well-demarcated tumor, frequently with areas of calcification.

Medulloblastoma

Medulloblastoma is the most common malignant tumor of childhood (4–8 years). It arises from embryonic tissue in the cerebellar vermis and may seed through the cerebrospinal fluid pathways to other parts of the cranium or the spinal cord.

Ependymoma

Ependymoma is the second most common tumor of childhood, although it is also found in individuals aged in their early 20s. It occurs throughout the ventricular system or the spinal canal, but is particularly common in the fourth ventricle and in the caudal part of the spinal cord. Frequently, it infiltrates surrounding tissues. Fourth-ventricle ependymomas usually present with symptoms of intermittent hydrocephalus, ataxia, vertigo, and vomiting.

Meninges
Meningioma

Meningioma is a benign tumor arising from the arachnoid that compresses rather than invades the neural tissues. Maximum incidence occurs between 40 and 60 years of age. It is most common in the sylvian region, the parasagittal surface of the parietal and frontal lobes, the olfactory grooves, the lesser wings of the sphenoid, the tuberculum sellae, the cerebellopontine angle, and the thoracic spinal cord. Imaging reveals a well-circumscribed lesion with occasional calcification. Surgery is a definite possibility in most of these patients.

Some meningiomas contain estrogen receptors, and may enlarge markedly in pregnancy.

145

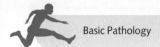

Nerve sheath cells
Neurofibroma
Neurofibroma is a benign, slow-growing tumor that commonly develops on the vestibular division of cranial nerve VIII (often misleadingly called an acoustic neuroma). It tends to present in midlife and is more common in females. Neurofibroma usually presents with sensorineural deafness, occasionally associated with tinnitus and vertigo. It may appear as part of the neurofibromatosis syndrome (most commonly type 2), when other tumors (particularly contralateral acoustic neuromas) should be sought.

Primary cerebral lymphoma (microglioma)
With the advent of HIV, and increasing numbers of immunosuppressed patients, this tumor is becoming more common. They are often periventricular, and may be multiple. Microgliomas are aggressive tumors, and account for up to 10% of central nervous system complications in AIDS patients.

Anterior pituitary gland
Pituitary adenoma
Pituitary adenoma is a benign tumor that presents with neurological or endocrinological symptoms. Large tumors usually present with headache, bitemporal hemianopia (from upward pressure on the optic chiasm), and occasionally hypopituitarism. Smaller tumors present with hyperprolactinemia and less commonly with acromegaly/gigantism, Cushing's syndrome, and thyrotoxicosis.

Other tissues
Tumors of other tissues can be summarized as:
- Blood vessels: hemangioblastoma.
- Germ cells: germinoma, teratoma.
- Microglia: primary brain lymphoma.
- Tumors of maldevelopmental origin: crangiopharyngioma, epidermoid/dermoid cyst, colloid cyst.
- Local extension from adjacent tumors: chordoma, glomus jugulare tumor.

Metastatic brain tumors
Metastatic brain tumors are around eight times more common than primary brain malignancies. Approximately 20% of patients dying with other tumors will have intracranial metastases, 25% of which are asymptomatic. The primary tumors are:
- 44% bronchus.
- 10% breast.
- 7% genitourinary.
- 6% bowel.
- 3% skin (melanoma).
- 30% others.

Presenting features are similar to those of the primary brain tumors, but the lesions are often multiple. On CT or MRI they have a round, well-circumscribed appearance, often with surrounding edema.

Investigations of brain tumors
Investigations are aimed to identify the presence of the tumor, its anatomical site, and its pathology with:
- Imaging (computed tomography, magnetic resonance imaging, angiography).
- Biopsy.

Treatment
Treatment depends on many factors, mainly the type, site, and stage of the tumor, and includes:
- Symptomatic: analgesia, steroids (to reduce cerebral edema), anticonvulsants.
- Specific: surgery, radiotherapy, chemotherapy.

Prognosis
The great majority of patients with cerebral tumors have a limited life expectancy, with a median survival of a few months. More benign tumors allow survival for many years.

Effects of systemic cancer on the central nervous system
These include:
- Direct invasion from adjacent structures.
- Metastatic disease.
- Nonmetastatic "remote effect" (paraneoplastic syndromes).
- Immunologically mediated:
  ○ Cerebellar dysfunction.
  ○ Visual dysfunction.
  ○ Sensory neuropathy.
  ○ Opsoclonus.
- Lambert–Eaton myasthenic syndrome.
- Limbic encephalitis.
- Others (opportunistic infections, dermatomyositis, inappropriate antidiuretic hormone secretion).

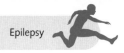

Epilepsy

An epileptic seizure (fit) is a paroxysmal alteration in nervous system activity that is time limited and causes a clinically detectable event. The types of epileptic seizure are shown in Fig. 11.16.

Epilepsy is a condition in which more than one seizure has occurred, in the absence of abnormal metabolic states (most individuals will develop seizures if they are sufficiently hyponatremic). Incidence is greatest in early and late life, with a prevalence of approximately 0.5%.

Febrile convulsions in childhood are not classed as epilepsy, although, if prolonged, these may predispose to epilepsy in later life.

Epilepsy is a clinical diagnosis and the patient is often normal on examination; therefore, a careful history is vital. It is particularly useful to obtain a history from a witness to the seizure.

A patient who has had a seizure with loss of consciousness may remember feeling odd (e.g., odd smells, metallic taste) before the event (the aura), and may remember feeling confused, disorientated, and sleepy afterwards (the postictal phase), but will have no memory of the seizure itself. Surprisingly, perhaps, tongue-biting and urinary incontinence are infrequently seen.

Risk of another seizure within 1 year of the first is 40%, rising to 50% within 3 years.

Status epilepticus is defined as seizures occurring in series with no recovery of consciousness, or a seizure lasting more than 30 minutes. It constitutes a medical emergency as there is a high risk of brain damage and death.

Partial (focal) epilepsy

Focal epilepsy may arise from an intracerebral structural defect, causing motor or sensory symptoms localized to one body part, which may then spread to adjacent areas as the electrical activity spreads to contiguous regions of the cortex (e.g., jacksonian seizure). These are simple partial seizures. Sometimes, no underlying structural defect can be found.

Complex partial seizures usually arise in the temporal lobe. They are called "complex" because they are associated with disturbance of consciousness.

Seizures arising in the medial temporal lobe may produce disturbances of smell and taste, visual hallucinations, and a sense of déjà vu. These may evolve to a tonic–clonic seizure (secondary generalization). Weakness following the event may occur for minutes or hours (Todd's paresis).

Primary generalized epilepsy

Any of the seizure types indicated in Fig. 11.16 may occur in one patient. In a generalized tonic–clonic seizure, the tonic ("increased tone") phase is a sudden tonic contraction of muscles usually with upward eye deviation. The clonic ("with clonus-type activity") phase follows. Initial EEG changes are often bilateral. This condition usually has its onset in childhood. Absence (or petit mal) attacks usually

Types of epileptic seizure	
primary generalized epilepsy	absence seizures; primary generalized tonic–clonic seizures; others; myoclonic, atypical absences; tonic, clonic, and atonic seizures
partial (focal) epilepsy ± secondary generalization	simple partial seizure (without loss of consciousness), complex partial seizures (with disturbed consciousness)
secondary generalized epilepsy	due to underlying generalized cerebral abnormality
epilepsy due to underlying focal or metabolic cause	primary intracranial lesions (tumor, stroke, infections, trauma), metabolic (hypoglycemia, hypomagnesemia, liver failure), drugs (and most in overdose), drug withdrawal (alcohol, benzodiazepines), toxins (alcohol, carbon monoxide)

Fig. 11.16 Types of epileptic seizure.

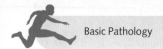
consist of a brief interruption of activity, sometimes with complex motor activity (such as fumbling with clothes), but without collapse. EEG during this event shows a three-per-second spike-and-wave activity (see Chapter 16).

Epilepsy syndromes

Certain conditions classified as epilepsy syndromes include clinical and EEG manifestations. These include:

- Benign childhood epilepsy with centrotemporal spikes.
- Lennox–Gastaut syndrome.
- Infantile spasms: characteristic brief episodes with shock-like flexion of arms, head, and neck and drawing up of the knees (called a salaam attack). It is associated with progressive mental handicap.
- Juvenile myoclonic epilepsy: a familial late childhood onset disease, with myoclonic jerks, tonic–clonic seizures ± absence seizures, with typical interictal EEG.

Pseudoseizures

Pseudoseizures (simulated seizures) occur in up to 20% of patients referred for "intractable epilepsy." They may occur in association with real epilepsy or psychological disturbance.

Prolactin levels may be useful in determining whether a seizure was real or simulated. In all complex and partial seizures (except absences), prolactin levels show an immediate rise, which the patient cannot simulate.

Investigation

This includes EEG—note that approximately 50% are normal and this does not disprove the diagnosis. Computed tomography, and/or magnetic resonance imaging in adult-onset seizures, with further investigation as appropriate to the individual.

Blood tests to identify reversible causes, along with a toxic screen and electrocardiogram (to identify long Q-T syndromes) are important in all patients.

Treatment

First seizures are often not treated but, unless seizures are years apart, most neurologists would treat after the second event. There are a wide range of antiepileptic medications, and choice depends mostly on seizure type. A major reason for differentiating partial from generalized seizures is that different drugs are effective for each. Some patients with suitable seizure activity may benefit considerably from surgical removal of an epileptogenic focus on a temporal lobe. Note that, in 70% of patients, epilepsy eventually remits, and trials of treatment withdrawal should be considered at an appropriate time.

Epilepsy and driving.
First seizure/solitary seizure.
- One year off driving (seizure-free) with medical review before restarting. If another seizure occurs during this time, the patient must wait a year from that seizure before review.

Loss of consciousness without known cause.
- As above.

Seizures during sleep.
- After one seizure, regulations as above. If all attacks for at least 3 years have been during sleep, and the patient has never had an awake attack, driving is allowed.

Withdrawal of antiepileptic medication.
- Advise not to drive (but not a legal obligation on the patient's part) for 6 months from time of withdrawal. Clearly, if further seizures occur, the above regulations apply.

Antiepileptic drugs
Phenytoin

Phenytoin reduces the spread of a seizure. Electroencephalogram recordings show that it does not stop the "spiking" at a focus and so it does not prevent the onset of an epileptic discharge, but stops it from involving other areas. It blocks voltage-gated

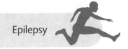

Na$^+$ channels and has a higher affinity for channels in the inactivated state. This state is prolonged, preventing the channel from opening, which stops the neuron from firing rapidly. The block is use-dependent as, at higher frequencies, more channels are cycling through the inactivated state. This allows selectivity of action, as the phenytoin block is more likely to occur in neurons in a seizure focus.

Oral absorption is variable and phenytoin is metabolized in the liver by an enzyme system that is saturated at therapeutic doses and, as such, shows dose-dependent kinetics. This means that, at certain doses, the serum concentration can rise rapidly to toxic levels as there is only a limited capacity to metabolize it. Because patients will vary in the doses that saturate their enzyme system, the therapeutic regime starts with low doses and then increases, with careful monitoring of serum phenytoin.

The side effects of phenytoin are:
- Vertigo and cerebellar signs—ataxia, dysarthria, nystagmus.
- At high doses, sedation and interference with cognitive functions.
- Collagen effects—gum hypertrophy and coarsening of facial features.
- Allergic reactions—rash, hepatitis, lymphadenopathy.
- Hematological effects—megaloblastic anemia.
- Endocrine effects—hirsutism.
- Teratogenesis—may cause congenital malformations (cleft palate).

Phenytoin has many drug interactions, mainly because it induces the hepatic P$_{450}$ oxidase system, increasing the metabolism of oral contraceptives, anticoagulants, dexamethasone, and pethidine. It is used for all types of epilepsy except absence seizures.

Carbamazepine

The mechanism of action of carbamazepine is the same as for phenytoin:
- It is well absorbed orally, with a long half-life (25–60 hours) when first given.
- Its side-effect profile is really limited to the nervous system, with ataxia, nystagmus, dysarthria, vertigo, and sedation. Similar to phenytoin, it is a strong enzyme inducer, causing similar interactions, and induces its own metabolism, which is why its half-life decreases if taken regularly.

- It is used as first-line treatment for partial seizures, and second-line for generalized seizures.

Sodium valproate

Sodium valproate has two mechanisms of action:
- As for phenytoin.
- It increases GABA content and GABA action, although this has no clear explanation.

It is well absorbed orally, has a half-life of 10–15 hours, and has much fewer side effects than other anticonvulsants, with the main problems being tremor, weight gain, hair thinning, and ankle swelling. Rarely, it can cause hepatic failure (check liver function tests regularly) and may be teratogenic. It interacts with other central nervous system depressants (e.g., alcohol), potentiating their effects. It is used as first-line treatment for generalized seizures.

Ethosuximide

The mechanism of action of ethosuximide is unknown. It is used only for absence seizures, as it may make tonic–clonic attacks worse. Its side effects are nausea, loss of appetite, and mood swings.

Vigabatrin (γ-vinyl-GABA)

Vigabatrin is an irreversible inhibitor of GABA transaminase and so reduces the metabolism of GABA. This means that more GABA is available for release. It is used as an adjunct to other therapies that do not adequately control a patient's epilepsy.

Its side effects are drowsiness, dizziness, depression, and visual hallucinations, and it is contraindicated if patients have a history of psychiatric problems. Abrupt withdrawal leads to rebound seizures. It can be retinotoxic, causing loss of peripheral visual field. Its use should be confined to specialist practice.

Phenobarbitone

Phenobarbitone is a barbiturate and has two anticonvulsant actions:
- It binds to the GABA$_A$ receptor, potentiating the effect of normal GABA release.
- It reduces glutamate-mediated excitation.

Its main side effect is sedation which, together with the fatal central nervous system depression that it causes in overdose, limits its use clinically.

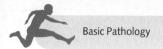
Phenobarbitone also causes cerebellar signs and is an enzyme inducer.

This is another drug to be used only in specialist practice.

Benzodiazepines

Benzodiazepines potentiate the normal effect of GABA binding.

Their side effects are sedation and they may cause an increase in the requirements for anticonvulsant drugs. They are used primarily in status epilepticus.

Treatment of status epilepticus

This is a medical emergency. Always consider whether the patient is pregnant, as it may be an eclamptic seizure which will only be cured by delivery of the baby. Otherwise, correct reversible causes (give a glucose infusion, and replace fluids). The initial treatment is with benzodiazepines (lorazepam or diazepam) ± phenytoin. If these therapies do not stop seizure activity, an anesthetist is required to supervise the administration of a barbiturate such as phenobarbitone.

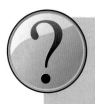

- What types of cerebral edema do you know? How may they be treated?
- How would you diagnose hydrocephalus?
- Describe the different neural tube defects you know.
- List five complications of skull fractures.
- Explain the mechanism of ischemic stroke. What risk factors do you know?
- What is the different pathology caused by rupture of Charcot–Bouchard and berry aneurysms?
- Name the three most common pathogens which cause acute bacterial meningitis. How would you diagnose the condition?
- Describe the classical features and symptoms of multiple sclerosis.
- Name three pathological changes in the brain tissue seen in Alzheimer's disease.
- Discuss the neurological complications of alcoholism.
- Which cancers metastasize to the brain? How would you identify their presence?
- What is the threshold for treating epilepsy? What would be your first-line treatment and emergency management of status epilepticus?

12. Pathology of the Peripheral Nerves and Muscle

In this chapter, you will learn about:
- Hereditary forms of neuropathy.
- Traumatic damage to nerves.
- Inflammatory neuropathies.
- Infectious causes of a neuropathy.
- Metabolic and toxic neuropathies.
- Neurocutaneous syndromes.
- Muscle diseases.
- Diseases of the neuromuscular junction.

Hereditary neuropathies

Hereditary motor and sensory neuropathies (HMSNs)

These include all inherited neuropathies that affect both the motor and sensory peripheral nerves. The incidence is approximately 1 : 2500. Classification of these diseases is changing as molecular genetic defects are discovered. No treatments are yet available, but much can be done in terms of helping the patient overcome his or her disability. Characteristic features include:
- Distal wasting and weakness (giving "inverted champagne-bottle legs").
- Areflexia.
- Pes cavus.
- Claw toes.
- Distal sensory loss.

HMSN I

This is also still called type 1, or hypertrophic (describing the histological appearance of the nerves) Charcot–Marie–Tooth (CMT) disease. It is usually autosomal dominant.

Charcot–Marie–Tooth disease is also known as peroneal muscular atrophy, referring to the wasting pattern in the legs.

Because myelin genes appear to be affected, it makes sense that this is a "demyelinating neuropathy," and nerve conduction velocities are slow. The disease usually presents in childhood or early teenage life with foot drop and leg weakness. Symptoms vary greatly: up to 20% of those affected are significantly disabled as adults, but a similar proportion are asymptomatic.

HMSN II

This is also still called type 2, or neuronal CMT syndrome. This is an "axonal" neuropathy (i.e., with relatively preserved nerve conduction velocity, but small motor and sensory action potentials). It is usually autosomal dominant, in some cases linked to c1. Presentation is similar to HMSN I, but wasting may be a more prominent feature.

HMSN III

This is also called Déjerine–Sottas disease. It is more severe, presenting in infancy. Recent molecular discoveries indicate that these cases may be "severe HMSN I."

- HMSN I is a demyelinating neuropathy with slow conduction velocities.
- HMSN II is an axonal neuropathy with near-normal conduction velocities.
- HMSN III presents like an early-onset, severe HMSN I.

Hereditary sensory neuropathy

This is a rare autosomal recessive or dominant condition that usually presents in childhood. Loss of pain occurs (predominantly) in the hands and feet. Charcot joint deformities and neuropathic ulcers of the feet also appear.

An osteoarthritic joint that has become grossly disorganized due to loss of pain sensation is known as a Charcot joint.

Hereditary sensory and autonomic neuropathy

There are five forms of hereditary sensory and autonomic neuropathies that are recognized. Their features are shown in Fig. 12.1.

Traumatic neuropathies

Trauma to a nerve causes weakness or numbness in the area supplied by that nerve, although sensory nerve injuries tend to cause symptoms and signs in an area smaller than that which the nerve supplies, owing to overlap in sensory territories. Trauma may partially or completely disrupt the nerve's function. Types of nerve injury are given in Fig. 12.2. Axons regenerate at a rate of 1.0–1.5 mm/day.

Compression neuropathy
Carpal tunnel syndrome

Carpal tunnel syndrome is common, especially in women. It is caused by pressure on the median nerve as it passes deep to the flexor retinaculum at the wrist. Initial symptoms are pain and tingling in the median nerve territory (most commonly the index and middle fingers), characteristically at night, causing the patient to shake the hand over the side of the bed for relief. Sometimes the pain shoots up the arm from the wrist. Signs may be absent initially. With time, median nerve innervated muscles, especially abductor pollicis brevis, may become weak and wasted and sensory signs may be found (Fig. 12.3).

Tinel's sign (tapping over the wrist) and Phalen's test (flexing the wrist for a minute) may reproduce symptoms, but a good history is the key to diagnosis. Predisposing factors for carpal tunnel syndrome are given in Fig. 12.4. The diagnosis may be confirmed with nerve conduction studies.

Treatment may be nonsurgical (wrist splints in slight extension, or local steroid injection) or surgical (division of the flexor retinaculum leading to decompression).

"Saturday night" palsy

"Saturday night" palsy is caused by compression of the radial nerve, especially if an arm is draped over a chair for some hours. It may also occur with fractures of the humerus (as the radial nerve runs in the spiral groove). Wrist drop and weakness of finger and thumb extension occur, but not usually sensory loss. Patients generally recover spontaneously in a few months.

Classification of HSANs	
Condition	Clinical features
HSAN I	Dominant inheritance. Absence of pain and temperature sensation (particularly distal). Charcot's joints and mutilation of feet common. Autonomic involvement rare.
HSAN II	Recessive inheritance. Combination of large and small fiber loss. Sensory loss is worse distally. Anhydrosis, areflexia, and mutilation of extremities occur. Blood pressure and sexual function normal.
HSAN III	"Riley–Day syndrome"—recessive. May present in neonates with hypothermia and vomiting crises. Pain and temperature insensitivity, areflexia, and autonomic crises in adults (postural hypotension, hypertension, sweating, etc.)
HSAN IV	Congenital sensory neuropathy with anhydrosis. Associated with mental retardation
HSAN V	Congenital absence of pain sensation without anhydrosis. Purely affects Aδ fibers

Fig. 12.1 Classification of the hereditary sensory and autonomic neuropathies (HSANs).

Fig. 12.2 Types of nerve injury, their effects, and potential for recovery.

Types of nerve injury		
Injury	**Extent**	**Effect**
Neurapraxia	Transient block. No structural damage. Usually compression of nerve is the cause	No degeneration of nerve fibers. Temporary disruption to nerve function which recovers fully
Axonotmesis	Rupture of nerve fiber within intact sheath. Prolonged pressure or crushing is a cause	Wallerian degeneration. Nerves regrow within sheath. Effects on function may be severe but complete recovery is usual
Neurotmesis	Complete section of nerve	Wallerian degeneration. Paralysis/sensory loss are complete. Regeneration may be slow and incomplete.

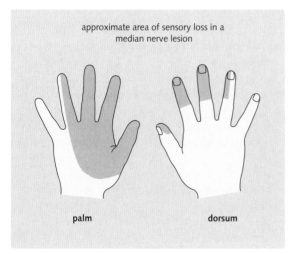

approximate area of sensory loss in a median nerve lesion

palm   dorsum

Fig. 12.3 Approximate area of sensory loss in a median nerve lesion.

Predisposing factors for carpal tunnel syndrome
arthritis of the wrist obesity pregnancy hypothyroidism and acromegaly repetitive wrist movements (washing floors, vibrating tools) hereditary neuropathy with liability to pressure palsies (HNPP)
But it is usually idiopathic!

Fig. 12.4 Predisposing factors for carpal tunnel syndrome.

Ulnar nerve compression

This usually occurs at the elbow (in the groove of the medial epicondyle), particularly during general anesthesia, with the use of crutches, and secondary to previous elbow injury. It can also occur in the cubital tunnel (the fibrous band between the heads of flexor carpi ulnaris). Symptoms include pain and paresthesias along the medial aspect of the forearm and numbness in the little and ring fingers, similar to that experienced when hitting your "funny bone." There may be wasting and weakness of ulnar-innervated small hand muscles, especially the first dorsal interosseous muscle. If the branch to flexor digitorum profundus is affected (in lesions above the cubital tunnel), there will also be weakness of flexion of the distal interphalangeal joint. The main complaint of patients is that they cannot grip objects effectively.

Treatment involves avoiding unnecessary trauma to the nerve (no leaning on the elbows) and sometimes surgery.

Meralgia paresthetica

This is a syndrome of tingling, pain, and numbness on the anterolateral surface of the thigh caused by compression of the lateral cutaneous nerve of the thigh under the lateral end of the inguinal ligament. It is more common in the obese, in pregnancy, and with very tight trousers.

Nerve roots damaged with cervical spondylosis			
Nerve root	Sensory supply	Motor supply	Reflexes
C5	Lateral arm and forearm	Shoulder abduction, elbow flexion	Biceps and supinator
C6	Lateral wrist and lateral hand	Elbow flexion	
C7	Middle finger	Elbow extension, finger flexion and extension	Triceps (with C8)

Fig. 12.5 Nerve roots commonly damaged with cervical spondylosis.

Treatment, other than weight reduction and reconsideration of wardrobe, is unnecessary.

Cervical spondylosis

Cervical spondylosis is a degenerative condition of the vertebral column and intervertebral disks, which is uncommon in patients aged under 50 years. It may cause compressive injuries of cervical roots as they pass through their foramina. The roots of C5, C6, and C7 are commonly affected. The symptoms are shown in Fig. 12.5.

Avulsions

Avulsion of the spinal roots is generally caused by severe traumatic injury. The most common area is brachial avulsions, but lumbosacral avulsions can occur. Two examples are:

- Erb's palsy: caused by avulsion of C5 and C6 roots because of pressure on the shoulder, usually after motorcycle accidents or, in babies, after forceps delivery. The shoulder cannot be abducted and the elbow cannot be flexed, therefore the arm hangs limply with the wrist flexed.
- Klumpke paralysis: avulsion of C8 and T1, usually occurring when the arm is pulled forcibly upward (particularly due to birth trauma). Loss of function affects the small muscles of the hand and the long finger flexors and extensors. This leads to a disabling claw hand deformity and may be associated with Horner's syndrome.

The characteristic deformity seen with Erb's palsy is known as the "waiter's tip" position. The arm is held straight, with the hand held palm upward, facing backwards.

Lacerations

Penetrating injury and fracture may lacerate a nerve, causing loss of function in the territory it supplies.

- Ulnar nerve: usually at the elbow, causing signs as above.
- Median nerve: with fractures in the arm, resulting in weakness of forearm flexors, flexor digitorum profundus (the patient cannot flex the distal interphalangeal joint of his forefinger) and, commonly, abductor pollicis brevis, together with sensory loss, as shown in Fig. 12.3. Note that a compression (between the two heads of pronator teres) or traumatic injury affecting the anterior interosseous nerve causes loss of flexion of the distal interphalangeal joints of the thumb, index finger, and sometimes middle finger, without sensory loss.
- Radial nerve: with fractures of the shaft of the humerus, causing a similar picture to Saturday night palsy.
- Femoral nerve: femoral artery cannulation may rarely result in damage.
- Sciatic nerve: may be damaged with fractures of the femur and pelvis, misplaced intramuscular injections, or penetrating injury.

Inflammatory neuropathies

Guillain–Barré syndrome (GBS)

This is a clinical syndrome caused by an acute peripheral neuropathy, affecting motor more than sensory nerves, and in most cases following infection. The incidence is approximately 1 : 50 000. Following the illness, 20% of patients remain so disabled that they are unable to work after a year, and 5% die. By definition, the illness progresses for less than 4 weeks. Approximately 70% of the patients recall a preceding diarrheal illness or upper respiratory tract infection a few days or weeks before neurological signs develop. These are most commonly *Campylobacter* (30% of cases) or CMV (10% of cases).

In most cases, there is inflammation and demyelination, hence the alternative name "acute inflammatory demyelinating polyradiculopathy" (AIDP). In approximately 5% of cases, the same clinical picture (i.e., syndrome) may be produced by an acute motor or acute motor and sensory axonal neuropathy (AMAN and AMSAN), where the brunt of the injury falls on the axons primarily, and the potential for spontaneous recovery may be less.

The clinical features are:
- Development of symptoms over days or weeks.
- Bilateral flaccid weakness (and later wasting) of proximal and distal limb muscles.
- Loss of tendon reflexes.
- Progression of weakness in some cases to affect the respiratory and bulbar (speech and swallowing) muscles.
- Burning pains and numbness, but often without sensory signs.

Important complications include:
- Respiratory failure and associated respiratory infections.
- Cardiac arrhythmias.
- Labile blood pressure and postural hypotension.
- Pressure sores.
- Anxiety and depression.

Investigations:
- In AIDP, in particular, nerve conduction studies show prolonged distal motor latencies in the upper and lower limbs. Slowing of conduction velocities is a late sign, and may not be seen at all. Action potentials are often reduced.
- Cerebrospinal fluid protein is usually raised (up to 5 g/dL), but the cell count is normal.

The Miller–Fisher syndrome is a variant of GBS with:
- An eye movement disorder caused by cranial nerve III, IV, or VI palsies.
- Cerebellar ataxia.
- Areflexia.

Management
Management involves avoidance of complications, by regular measurement of the vital capacity (deterioration may be rapid; the patient may require ventilation only hours after symptoms begin), constant electrocardiogram recording, and careful nursing. Patients may require long stays in intensive care, with 25% requiring respiratory support. Plasma exchange and intravenous immunoglobulin are equally effective at hastening recovery. Pain may be a prominent feature—good physiotherapy and nonsteroidal anti-inflammatory drugs are helpful.

The disease ultimately is self-limiting, with remyelination of axons within a matter of weeks.

Differential diagnosis of Guillain–Barré syndrome
Neuropathies:
- Porphyria.
- Acute heavy metal poisoning.
- Diphtheria.
- Vasculitis.
- HIV-related neuropathy.

Anterior horn cell:
- Poliomyelitis.

Central nervous system:
- Cord compression.
- Transverse myelopathy.
- Brainstem infarction.

Neuromuscular:
- Myasthenia gravis.
- Botulism.

Muscular:
- Periodic paralysis.
- Acute polymyositis.

Chronic inflammatory demyelinating polyradiculopathy (CIDP)
CIDP has a similar pathology to GBS, but it follows a relapsing–remitting course, with more slowly progressive onset of signs.

The condition responds in 80% of cases to steroids, intravenous immunoglobulin, and plasma exchange.

Paraproteinemic neuropathy
Paraproteinemic neuropathy is associated with:
- Benign monoclonal gammopathy (of undetermined significance)—demyelinating neuropathy with immunoglobulin M and immunoglobulin G paraproteins.

- Multiple myeloma (especially osteosclerotic)—neuropathy in 5% of cases, typically mixed sensory and motor.
- Solitary plasmacytoma—as for myeloma, often responsive to radiation or surgery to remove the primary tumor.
- Waldenström's macroglobulinemia.

Infectious neuropathies

Postinfectious neuropathies

These include:

- Guillain–Barré syndrome.
- Diphtheria: progressive peripheral neuropathy caused by the exotoxin, may occur a few weeks after the acute febrile illness. Supportive treatment until recovery is necessary.
- Lyme disease (Bannwarth's syndrome): rare in developed countries. A Guillain–Barré-type syndrome may occur some weeks later. Treatment of the acute illness is with benzylpenicillin; the subsequent neuropathy recovers gradually.

Infectious neuropathies

They include:

- **Leprosy**: common in southern Asia and Africa. Causes a patchy peripheral neuropathy (primarily sensory loss) with hypopigmented, anesthetic skin lesions and thickened nerves. Diagnosis is by skin or nerve biopsy; the acid-fast bacilli are seen within the tissue.
- **Tetanus**: caused by infection of a wound by *Clostridium tetani*. Days to weeks later, rigidity and pain in voluntary muscles occur, with difficulty opening the jaw (trismus), facial stiffness (risus sardonicus), dysphagia, back stiffness, hyperextension, and respiratory difficulty. Spasms may be strong enough to cause vertebral crush fractures, and may lead to exhaustion and respiratory failure. Treatment includes debriding the initial wound, benzylpenicillin, human antitetanus immunoglobulin, and good supportive care in a quiet environment (because stimulation may induce spasms). Diazepam may be used to control spasms.
- **Botulism**: caused by ingestion of *Clostridium botulinum*. A neurotoxin may cause symptoms because of cholinergic blockade. Hours to days later, lower motor neuron and autonomic symptoms may occur, generally beginning with blurred vision and diplopia. Flaccid weakness and paralysis (particularly of the laryngeal and pharyngeal muscles) spreading to include respiratory muscles. This may mimic myasthenia gravis or Guillain–Barré syndrome. Antitoxin treats the acute infection but the mainstay of management is good supportive care whilst awaiting recovery.
- **Herpes simplex** (type 2) virus: may cause lumbosacral radiculopathy.
- **Herpes zoster virus** or "shingles": or a reactivation of latent herpes zoster which has remained dormant in the dorsal root ganglia since an attack of chickenpox in earlier life. It may occur in normal people, but is more common in the immunosuppressed (especially those with hematological malignancies and AIDS). A dermatomal vesicular rash is usually present. Symptoms caused by peripheral nerve involvement include pain, then numbness in the area of the rash, flaccid weakness in the root distribution of the rash, which may then spread (and may even progress to Guillain–Barré syndrome). Intravenous acyclovir is the treatment for all neurologically serious complications of herpes virus infections.
- **HIV**: may present with a variety of neurological manifestations. Acute complications include mild viral meningitis at the time of seroconversion, meningoencephalitis, facial palsy, peripheral neuropathy, dorsal root ganglionitis (acute ataxic neuropathy), transverse myelitis, and polymyositis. Chronic neurological problems include vacuolar myelopathy, peripheral neuropathy, and AIDS dementia complex. These patients are also susceptible to opportunistic infections such as: CMV radiculopathy, cryptococcal meningitis, toxoplasmosis (cerebral abscesses), progressive multifocal leucoencephalopathy, tuberculous meningitis, and atypical mycobacteria. In addition, tumors such as primary central nervous system B-cell lymphoma may occur.

Metabolic and toxic neuropathies

Diabetes mellitus

Diabetes is the most common cause of neuropathy. It is more common with poorly controlled diabetics

The periodic paralyses	
Hyperkalemic periodic paralysis	Hypokalemic periodic paralysis
sodium-channel mutations, chromosome 17	calcium-channel mutations, chromosome 1
autosomal recessive	autosomal dominant
occurs with rest after exercise and may have periocular myotonia	occurs after meals and with rest after exercise
short attacks of weakness (about 1 hour) which may be aborted by exercise at onset	weakness for several hours

Fig. 12.7 The potassium channel periodic paralyses. Note that the presentations are often identical, and the conditions cannot often be differentiated clinically.

Myasthenia gravis is associated with acetylcholine-receptor antibodies at the neuromuscular junction. Both immunological and genetic factors appear to be important in its pathogenesis.

The condition is associated with lymphoid hyperplasia and tumors of the thymus. Weakness may respond to surgical thymic removal, especially in young patients with a short history. Otherwise, treatment is with immunosuppression and with anticholinesterases.

Lambert–Eaton myasthenic syndrome

This is characterized by weakness that is initially lessened with exercise. It is a rare disorder that is more common in men. It is caused by an autoimmune destruction of presynaptic voltage-gated calcium channels at the NMJ, causing a reduction in the amount of acetylcholine released.

Disorders of neuromuscular transmission
Myasthenia gravis

The prevalence of myasthenia gravis is approximately 1:20000. Women are affected twice as frequently as men. The condition is characterized by fatiguable weakness of periocular, facial, and proximal muscles [i.e., it worsens with exercise, and usually gets worse as the day goes on (diurnal)].

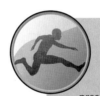

- Lambert–Eaton myasthenic syndrome is associated in up to 60% of cases with a small-cell lung carcinoma. Patients presenting this way should be fully investigated.

- Describe the key clinical features of Charcot–Marie–Tooth disease.
- What are the features of carpal tunnel syndrome. What clinical tests could you do to make the diagnosis?
- Describe the different ways in which a nerve may be traumatized.
- Give an example of a postinfectious neuropathy, and discuss its sequelae.
- What are the possible consequences of diabetic neuropathy?
- What is neurofibromatosis? How is it classified and diagnosed?
- Compare Duchenne and Becker muscular dystrophies.
- Describe the underlying abnormality in myasthenia gravis. How is it diagnosed and treated?

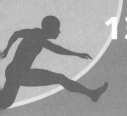

13. Higher Centers of the Central Nervous System

In this chapter, you will learn about:
- The functions of different areas of the cerebral cortex.
- Mechanisms of learning and memory.
- The limbic system and its functions.
- Cognition and cognitive impairment.
- Disorders of higher central nervous system function.
- Antiemetic drugs.
- General anesthetics.

Localization of function and behavior

Structural and functional asymmetry

There are structural differences between hemispheres.

The planum temporale (superior aspect of the temporal lobe lying within the lateral sulcus) is larger on the left side in the majority of individuals. Wernicke's area lies in the posterior part of the planum temporale, and speech comprehension is affected by damage to this area of the temporal lobe on the left, but not on the right. Along with the fact that the left side of the brain controls the right hand (dominant in most people), this has led to the concept of "left hemisphere dominance." A small but significant number of left-handed people have right-hemisphere speech.

The localization of functional areas has been experimentally demonstrated by:
- Positron emission tomography (PET) or functional magnetic resonance imaging of normal subjects performing a range of tasks.
- Wada test, where sodium amytal is injected into one carotid artery, which temporarily anesthetizes one hemisphere so that tasks can be processed only by the contralateral side. For example, injection of sodium amytal into the left carotid artery will temporarily block speech in most subjects.

Although the left and right hemispheres are connected through the corpus callosum, they carry out different functions. The evidence for this comes from:

- Patients with lesions localized to one hemisphere (e.g., patients who have aphasia following a left hemisphere stroke).
- Patients with severe grand mal epilepsy who have undergone sectioning of the corpus callosum (commissurotomy) to prevent spread of seizures.
- "Split-brain" animal studies, in which a commissurotomy has been carried out.

In a classical experiment on commissurotomy patients, subjects were presented with a picture of an apple solely within the right visual field. A patient would report seeing an apple, as might be expected. However, if the object was presented to the left visual field (and therefore to the right hemisphere), the patient reported seeing nothing. The patient had not lost his left visual field, as he was able to point to an apple, or to pick it out using tactile clues. In other words, a subject's right hemisphere could not name the object, but could identify it by nonverbal means. Split-brain experiments may not give us the whole story, as there is some evidence that the ability of a hemisphere to carry out a task may deteriorate after commissurotomy. However, in a simplified view, lateralization can be summarized:
- The left hemisphere is involved in intellectual reasoning and language.
- The right hemisphere is more concerned with spatial construction (including depth perception and the internal "map" of our surroundings) and emotion.

This will not be true for all patients, and the existence of commissural connections complicates this picture.

There is an element of plasticity in the location of function. In children who sustain damage to one hemisphere, the other can take over its functions so that there is no appreciable deficit. This is not the case in adults, as shown by the effects of a stroke.

Cortical localization

Different cortical regions perform different functions. This is because of their different input and output connections.

Regions within different lobes can be split up into functional units:

- Primary sensory or motor areas, which receive information from outside the brain or project outside the brain.
- Higher-order sensory or motor areas. These areas carry out further processing on information from one modality. For example, visual areas V2–V5 segregate information into the color, form, and motion channels. The supplementary motor area has a role in planning movements by integrating inputs from the prefrontal cortex, basal ganglia, and cingulate cortex.
- Association areas, where information from different modalities is brought together for processing that encompasses more than just vision, hearing, etc. (e.g., the posterior parietal cortex has a role in integrating visual information with somatic information to give an awareness of one's presence in space).

Frontal lobes

The frontal lobes have:

- An association area that plans sequences of responses, changes response patterns to fit current demands, and controls emotional states.
- Higher-order motor processing areas that have motor control functions for eye movements (the frontal eye fields) and speech (Broca's area on the dominant side).

Therefore frontal cortex damage can produce:

- Inability to organize responses to solve problems.
- An error pattern of "perseveration" in tasks where changes must be responded to. The Wisconsin card-sorting test is based on asking a subject to sort cards according to one rule (e.g., same color), and then the examiner changes the rule (e.g., to same pattern). The subject works out the new rule by feedback from the examiner about correct or incorrect card sorting. Perseveration occurs when subjects do not change from using a previously correct rule that has become incorrect.
- Personality changes occurring along emotional dimensions. Patients typically become more impulsive, aggressive, and subject to rapid changes in emotional state. This is referred to as disinhibition.
- Disordered eye movement scanning of a visual scene.

- Damage to Broca's area produces problems in speech production with hesitant, limited speech (described as "telegrammatic").
- Disordered working memory (with distractability).

It is rare for these patients to have insight into their condition.

Perseveration may be an important feature in dementia. When asked their name, patients may answer correctly, but subsequent (different) questions will elicit the same answer.

Temporal lobes

The temporal lobes have:

- Association areas that are involved in learning.
- Higher-order sensory areas involved in the comprehension of language (Wernicke's area) and visual object recognition.

The consequences of temporal damage are:

- Disorders in learning verbal information in left-sided lesions.
- Disorders in learning visuospatial information in right-sided lesions.
- Problems in understanding spoken and written language but no reduction in fluency of language production (receptive aphasia). This results in meaningless or irrelevant speech.
- Object agnosia, where patients cannot recognize objects from visual information but can do so from other modalities (e.g., touch).

Parietal lobes

The parietal lobes have:

- A primary sensory area receiving somatosensory information.
- A higher-order sensory area.
- An association area where many sensory modalities and motor inputs converge to build up a picture of how the body is positioned in the environment (incorporating attentional mechanisms) and how the environment is structured.

Damage can therefore produce:
- Lack of conscious sensation on one half of the body.
- Attentional deficits presenting as neglect (usually of the left half of space after a right-sided lesion).
- Inability to make voluntary eye movements and optic ataxia after bilateral parieto-occipital damage (Balint syndrome).
- Constructional apraxia, which is an inability to organize movement in space (seen with right-sided lesions). It is tested by attempting to copy a figure by drawing, typically interlocking pentagons.
- Disorders of spatial awareness (also mainly seen with right-sided lesions). This manifests as a defect in route finding (spatial navigation).
- Disorders of language (mainly with damage to the dominant parietal lobe, although the emotional content of speech is processed in the nondominant hemisphere.
- Agnosia—this is the inability to perceive objects normally. People with parietal damage may have astereognosia—an inability to recognize objects by touch. For example, they could not identify a particular coin by touch alone, without looking at the coins.

Each hemisphere represents the contralateral half of space in the parietal cortex. However, there is an unequal amount of space represented in each hemisphere. The left hemisphere represents only the right side of space. The right hemisphere represents the left and some of the right side of space. The right side of space is therefore slightly overrepresented. This means that lesions of the left parietal cortex will not severely affect processing of the right side of space because it is also being carried out to some extent in the right parietal cortex.

Right-sided lesions will produce more severe effects on the processing of the left half of space because it is analyzed entirely within the right hemisphere.

Learning and memory

Learning is the acquisition of new information. Memory is the retention of learned information, and can be divided into two basic parts:
- Declarative memory for facts (semantic memory, e.g., Austin is the capital of Texas) and events (episodic memory, e.g., I had a sandwich for lunch). This is easy both to acquire and to lose.
- Procedural memory for skills/behavior, which is hard to acquire and also hard to lose (even in profound loss of declarative memory, you never forget how to ride a bike).

Declarative memory can be split into three parts, as shown in Fig. 13.1:
- Sensory memory.
- Working memory.
- Long-term memory.

Sensory memory
Sensory memory is a store of all the sensory information that has just been processed. It is held in stores that are modality specific (e.g., visual stores, tactile stores) with a very high capacity, but that are limited in the time for which information can be held (fading after 0.5 sec).

There is no conscious access to sensory memory. Its function is in selective attention, filtering the inputs that will be consciously processed by working memory.

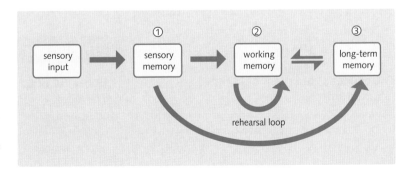

Fig. 13.1 The three-stage model of memory.

165

Working memory

Working memory contains the information that we are processing "right now" and we have conscious access to it. Inputs to working memory are from sensory memory or long-term memory.

- Its span (maximum capacity) is typically less than a dozen units of information (number, word, etc.).
- It functions as a push-down stack, so that new units of information displace the oldest units from the working memory store. Units are generally thought to be stored only for a few minutes at most.
- It has a visual store and a verbal store. Words are more likely to be coded by their acoustic properties than by semantic properties (what the words mean).

Long-term memory

Long-term memory is a collection of different types of memory that are grouped together by the nature of the information stored. As a general principle of long-term memory properties, these stores show unlimited capacity, but there are limitations in the capacity of the retrieval mechanism.

Distinctions between long-term memory and working memory
Studies of amnesia

In Wernicke–Korsakoff syndrome, the amnesia affects memory for events in adult life (sparing childhood memories) but patients have a preserved working memory span.

The serial position effect

After giving normal subjects a list of data, then asking them to recall the information freely in any order, the first and last units of information are preferentially recalled (the primacy and recency effects, respectively). After a delay before testing recall, the recency effect is lost. This suggests that working memory holds the most recently given data and that the first few units of information have made it into the long-term stores.

The coding strategy for holding verbal information

Working memory uses an acoustic strategy (evidence for this comes from error patterns made by normal subjects when recalling verbal information) whereas long-term memory stores verbal information in terms of meaning (typically, we can remember the "gist" of what people have said without recalling the actual words used).

Capacity for information

Working memory is limited in terms of the amount of information it holds and the time for which it is held. Long-term memory has an unlimited capacity for information and the information held has a much longer "shelf life." Over time, there is either gradual loss of storage space or, more likely, a diminished capacity to retrieve the information stored. Thus, we tend to get more forgetful as we get older.

Amnesia and localization of memory function

Amnesia is the loss of memory and/or the ability to learn, either caused by brain injury (organic amnesia) or for psychological reasons such as great stress (psychogenic amnesia).

- Retrograde amnesia is a loss of memory for things before the injury. Memories that have recently been transferred from the short-term to long-term stores may be more vulnerable to disruption.
- Anterograde amnesia is an inability to form new memories after injury.

Medial temporal lobe structures (e.g., the hippocampus and parahippocampal gyrus) have been implicated in memory function, and damage in these areas produces disruption of declarative memory, sparing procedural memory. This area receives highly processed information from association cortices and, as a possible cellular basis for memory, long-term potentiation (see below) has been recorded in cells in the hippocampus. Memory disruption may also occur after frontal and thalamic lesions.

The limbic system

Overview of the limbic system

The limbic system is a complex system of fiber tracts and gray matter. It is located on the medial aspect of each temporal lobe, encircling (limbus = border) the upper part of the brainstem.

- It serves as the "nervous system" for emotional feelings and behavior.
- It has extensive connections to both lower and higher parts of the central nervous system, which give the system an ability to integrate a wide variety of stimuli.
- It has connections with the hypothalamus to provide a substrate for a variety of nervous, hormonal, and visceral interactions.

The limbic system is in a position to influence both higher cognitive processes and lower homeostatic regulatory processes. Emotion, by its very nature, seems to bridge these two types of processing, requiring dimensions of thought and physical sensations. Memory plays a role in emotion, particularly in guiding behavioral responses to the environment, but the memory functions of the limbic system are not restricted to emotionally laden stimuli.

Although this picture of different functions may seem confusing, it highlights the areas to be aware of when dealing with patients who have suffered damage to these regions.

Structure of the limbic system

Fig. 13.2 shows the arrangement of limbic structures. We can consider the complicated connections of the limbic system as two simpler systems:

- A system primarily involved in learning and memory.
- A system involved with the processing of emotion, particularly its behavioral and endocrine aspects.

There are modulatory inputs from the reticular formation. The locus ceruleus sends a noradrenergic input and the raphe nuclei send a serotonergic input.

Hippocampal circuit

The hippocampal circuit runs from the medial temporal lobe (hippocampus and parahippocampal gyrus) to the mammillary bodies and thalamus, and is involved in learning and memory. The connections offer some guide as to how information flows in the circuit, as shown in Fig. 13.3.

There is some debate about the precise role of this circuit, particularly the hippocampus,

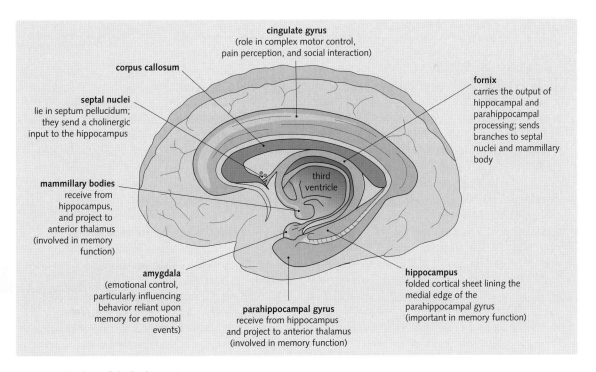

Fig. 13.2 Outline of the limbic system.

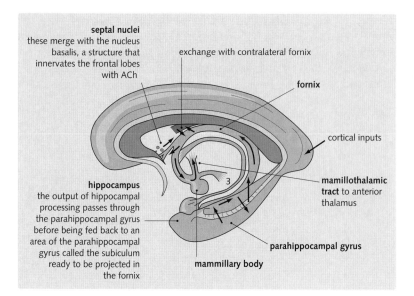

Fig. 13.3 Processing in the hippocampal circuit. To trace the pathway, start at the hippocampus and follow the arrows.

septal nuclei
these merge with the nucleus basalis, a structure that innervates the frontal lobes with ACh

exchange with contralateral fornix

fornix

cortical inputs

hippocampus
the output of hippocampal processing passes through the parahippocampal gyrus before being fed back to an area of the parahippocampal gyrus called the subiculum ready to be projected in the fornix

mamillothalamic tract to anterior thalamus

3

parahippocampal gyrus

mammillary body

parahippocampal gyrus, and mammillary bodies, but the following points are clear:

- Damage to the medial temporal lobe involving the hippocampus and parahippocampal gyrus (e.g., after herpes simplex encephalitis) produces a profound defect in declarative memory acquisition. This leads to anterograde amnesia. Long-term memories are stored in the overlying cerebral cortex.

- The physiological properties of cells in the hippocampus allow them to give increased responses to certain patterns of input. This occurs via long-term potentiation, which is an increase in the efficacy of a synapse with repetitive stimulation. It is mediated by NMDA glutamate receptors, which are plentiful in the hippocampus. Repeated depolarization of the postsynaptic membrane causes an alteration in the NMDA receptor, allowing calcium to enter the cell. This causes protein kinase activation, and phosphorylation of the AMPA glutamate receptor (the receptor used under normal circumstances at glutamatergic synapses). The sequence of events is summarized in Fig. 13.4.

- Degeneration of the mammillary bodies occurs in Wernicke–Korsakoff syndrome, where a combination of alcohol abuse and thiamine deficiency results in a memory disorder with anterograde amnesia.

Alzheimer's disease is typified by the inability to form new memories, and is due to the deposition of neurofibrillary tangles and amyloid plaques in the parahipppocampal areas.

Amygdaloid circuit

This circuit is less clear in function, possibly as a result of its rather diffuse connections.

The amygdala is a collection of nuclei lying at the anterior tip of the medial temporal lobe just anterior to the hippocampus. Fig. 13.5 shows inputs to the amygdala. Its outputs are simply connections traveling to the sources of input (reciprocal connections), but the largest output is to the hypothalamus through the stria terminalis.

There are many potential functions for the amygdala, though no "unifying theory" has yet been proposed.

- Lesion experiments on animals examining the function of the lateral part of the amygdala suggest that this circuit is involved in governing behavior toward stimuli associated with reward (particularly food).

- When the amygdala is stimulated, patients report strong feelings of fear. There is an accompanying

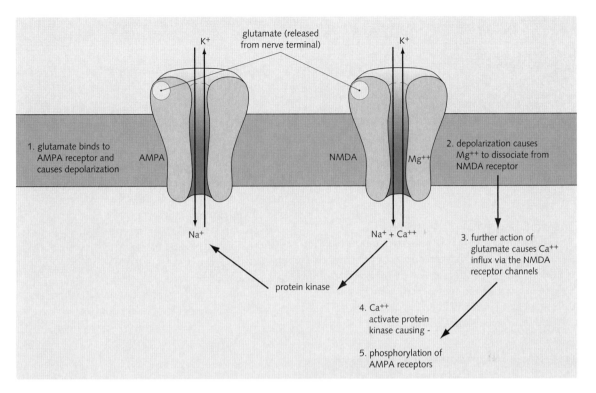

Fig. 13.4 Proposed mechanism of long-term potentiation.

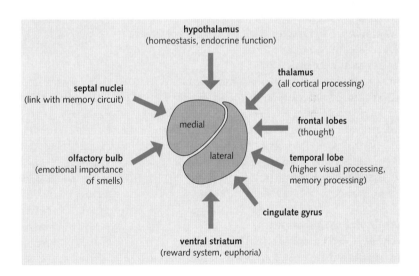

Fig. 13.5 Connections of amygdala.

sympathetic autonomic response. This has led to the theory that emotional reactions may be partly determined by activity in the amygdala. Lesions may cause impaired recognition of emotional facial expressions of other people. Ablation of the amygdala and hippocampus in monkeys produces the Klüver–Bucy syndrome, characterized by decreased emotionality, withdrawal, tendency to put everything in their mouths, and hypersexuality. Patients with temporal lobe epilepsy tend to show the opposite of these symptoms.

- The amygdala is implicated in learning, particularly the association of a stimulus and an emotional response.

The inability of autistic children to "read" the facial expressions of others has been used as evidence for there being damage in the amygdala. The social isolation that is characteristic of autism is more typical of cingulate damage.

The cingulate gyrus

The cingulate gyrus loops around the limbic system and lateral ventricles. It has a role in complex motor behavior, pain perception, and social interactions.

Patients with lesions in this area are typically socially isolated individuals, and may be so withdrawn as to be akinetic (not moving) and mute.

Cognitive development and degeneration

Cognitive development

Cognitive development in children is assessed by learning tests and by observation of their behavior. There are set "milestones" that children should have achieved by certain ages.

Many factors influence the rate of cognitive development and the level that individuals ultimately achieve. The chemical environment is crucial both *in utero* and in early childhood, as is nutritional status during this period. Depending on how cognitive function is assessed, the amount and quality of education will influence final performance.

Ability of the newborn

The newborn's cognitive abilities include:

- Auditory discrimination, as well as localization of the sound source. This is tested by observing head movements.
- Operant learning where, if certain responses are rewarded, babies will be more likely to make those responses.
- The production of smooth pursuit eye movements.
- Preferential interest in certain stimuli (e.g., human faces).

The newborn's motor capabilities are basic motor programs (e.g., reaching movements if body weight is supported).

The social behavior of the newborn is to interact with the primary caregiver by imitation of facial movements.

Motor changes

New motor abilities emerge in a set pattern, with the rate of appearance varying according to stimulation and encouragement of the child. Certain conditions (e.g., Down's syndrome) will adversely affect the attainment of these milestones.

Visual input is crucial to the natural development of reaching movements. Babies who are congenitally blind need special devices, such as echo locators, to develop appropriate reaching movements.

The fundamental changes in motor development as the child gets older are greater control over fine movements and greater fluidity in a series of movements.

Detetection of blindness (e.g., from congenital cataracts) and deafness in the newborn is essential.

Perceptual changes

Changes in perceptual ability involve learning how to interpret sensory information. One milestone is the development of depth perception shown by Gibson's visual cliff experiment. An infant is allowed to freely explore a table, part of which is transparent revealing a drop to floor level. In very young infants, there is no sign of fear to the apparent risk of falling. During the period of crawling, however, infants will not cross the visual cliff onto the transparent area.

The rate of acquisition of knowledge about the environment limits the development of perceptual abilities and will also affect attentional mechanisms.

Overall scheme of cognitive development: Piaget's theory
Sensorimotor stage: 0–2 years

Exploration of the environment occurs, and the child learns to distinguish themselves from it (the beginnings of self-awareness). This stage is also characterized by the development of object permanence, where infants understand that objects still exist when they can no longer perceive them (e.g., after removing them from the visual field). For Piaget, this was the basis of thought because it demonstrates that infants can hold representations of objects in their minds.

Preoperational stage: 2–7 years
Children at this stage are able to engage in symbolic play—using language and pictures to represent experiences. There is a decline in egocentricity—they can empathize with others.

Concrete operational thought: 7–11 years
This stage is characterized by the development of conservation, where children can appreciate that some aspects of objects remain the same, despite changes in appearance. This is displayed with the pencils test—two identical pencils are placed so that they have their bases and tips aligned. One is then moved relative to the other so that it looks longer than the other (if one ignores the fact that the bases have moved relative to each other). Children who conserve will not infer that, when the pencils have moved, one must be longer than the other. Children at this stage are capable of logical thought—seeing relationships between things and applying rules to new situations—but cannot undertake tasks involving abstract reasoning.

Formal operational thought: 11–15 years
At this stage, the ability of abstract reasoning develops.

Language acquisition
The process of language acquisition is not well understood, but current thinking is that there is a preprogrammed way of understanding language construction.

This inbuilt understanding of the workings of language allows rapid learning at a young age, no matter how that language is presented (i.e., learning and ease of use is the same for verbal and sign systems; deaf children learn sign language more quickly and use it in a far richer fashion than their hearing parents).

Children with delayed speech should have urgent investigation for hearing deficits, as language may be more difficult to acquire as the child gets older.

Cognitive degeneration
The aging brain
The gross changes in the brain include reductions in total volume, weight and size of gyri, and an increase in ventricular size. This is due to atrophy (i.e., the shrinkage of cells) along with nerve cell loss.

Neuronal death may be due to preprogramming, sensitivity to certain factors, or accumulated mutations.

Successful aging
A decline in mental function is not an inevitable consequence of aging. Compensatory sprouting of dendrites by remaining neurons can help to maintain the total number of synaptic connections. This process is called reactive synaptogenesis.

Reactive synaptogenesis explains why there is an increase in the length of dendrites in hippocampal granule cells between middle and old age. The mean dendritic length begins to fall back after 80 years, suggesting that there is a limit to how long this process can continue protecting against the effects of cell loss.

Dementia
Dementia has emerged as a modern disease, owing to increases in life expectancy. Of individuals aged over 65 years, 5% are severely demented.

The most common form of dementia is the Alzheimer type, where there is a cognitive decline affecting all aspects of cognition and personality (e.g., memory, attention, orientation, etc.). The neuronal pathology is characteristic, including:

- Disturbances of the cytoskeleton, called neurofibrillary tangles, composed of paired helical filaments of a protein called τ (tau), which is an abnormally phosphorylated form of a microtubule-associated protein.
- Extracellular deposits of protein rich in β-amyloid and apolipoprotein E, called senile plaques. The precursor of β-amyloid is a cell membrane protein acting as a protease inhibitor. Mutations in the gene coding for the precursor protein may be responsible for some of the familial cases of Alzheimer's disease.

There is a characteristic decrease in brain weight and cortical atrophy. There is marked loss of neurons, usually most prominent in the hippocampus, parahippocampal gyrus, and the frontal, anterior temporal, and parietal cortices (mainly affecting glutamatergic pyramidal neurons).

Cell loss also occurs in the basal forebrain complex, notably the basal nucleus (of Meynert), which gives rise to a diffuse acetylcholine projection to much of the neocortex, and the medial septal nuclei which give a diffuse cholinergic innervation to the hippocampus. Therapeutic strategies to increase acetylcholine release in the brain have had some limited success.

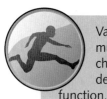 Vascular dementia (so-called multi-infarct dementia) is characterized by a stepwise deterioration in cognitive function.

Psychological aspects of aging

The normal changes in cognitive function begin at between 50 and 60 years of age and comprise:

- Reduction in the ability to perform problem-solving tasks, particularly if the problems are very novel or involve switching between different types of responses.
- Slowing of responses in certain cognitive tests, due to reductions in decision speed rather than motor function.
- Memory function decreases, affecting visual information more than verbal information, and recall more than recognition.
- Alterations of motor functions (particularly proprioceptive dysfunction, changes in gait, and muscle weakness).

Often, there are changes in social functioning, so-called disengagement behavior, where there is withdrawal from social contact. This may be caused by a lack of opportunity for social contact due to physical limitations on travel or financial limitations. As such, this may not represent a personality change, but may be a symptom of depression.

Mood changes after the age of 60 years typically include depression and anxiety as reactions against a perceived loss of a role in society, loss of social support, and bereavement. This should not be assumed to be "normal."

Pharmacology of higher central nervous system function

Anxiolytics and hypnotics

Anxiety is an exaggeration of a normal state with a cognitive component (unpleasant feelings of fear and restlessness) and an autonomic component (tachycardia, gastrointestinal upset, sweating). Anxiolytics reduce the symptoms of anxiety, whereas hypnotics enable people to sleep. This distinction is not clear-cut, particularly if anxiety is the main impediment to normal sleep.

Benzodiazepines

Benzodiazepines bind to-$GABA_A$ receptors (ligand-gated Cl^- channels), increasing their affinity for GABA (γ-aminobutyric acid). This increases the inhibitory effect of GABA on the postsynaptic cell.

Benzodiazepines have four main actions:
- Anxiolysis (both the cognitive and somatic symptoms).
- Sedation and sleep.
- Anticonvulsant.
- Reduction in voluntary muscle tone.

Their clinical uses are in anxiety states, preoperative sedation, status epilepticus, acute alcohol withdrawal, and sedation during endoscopy and bronchoscopy.

Their main side effects are:
- Psychomotor impairment and drowsiness.
- Incoordination, weakness, diplopia.
- Amnesia.
- Disinhibition (leading to inappropriate behaviors, including aggression).
- Dependence.

Fig. 13.6 shows the mechanism and site of action of benzodiazepines.

Dependence is shown after 4–6 weeks and is both psychological and physical. The withdrawal syndrome (in 30% of patients) comprises rebound anxiety and insomnia, tremors, and twitching. Withdrawal is more severe after taking a short-acting benzodiazepine.

In overdose, benzodiazepines alone will produce a long sleep but, particularly if alcohol is taken as well, the central nervous system depressant effects are potentiated and fatal respiratory depression can

effects, and mild extrapyramidal motor disturbance.
- Piperazine side chains (e.g., in fluphenazine) produce low sedation, mild autonomic effects, and strong extrapyramidal motor disturbance.

Thioxanthines and butyrophenones
These two groups of compounds have a similar profile to the piperazine group of phenothiazines, with low sedation, mild autonomic effects, and strong motor disturbance.
- Flupenthixol is a thioxanthine.
- Haloperidol is a butyrophenone.

Atypical neuroleptics
Drugs that have antipsychotic action but produce less intense motor side effects are termed "atypical."

Clozapine has 5-HT, α-adrenergic, and histamine blocking effects. It has minimal central antidopaminergic activity, and therefore produces few extrapyramidal side effects. The main risk with its use is agranulocytosis, and patients need close monitoring. It is particularly useful in those who are refractory to classical antipsychotics, or who experience extreme side effects.

Other drugs that are gaining popularity due to their favorable side-effect profile include:
- Risperidone.
- Olanzepine.
- Quetiapine.
- Amisulpride.

Overall neuroleptic side-effect profile
As well as the autonomic, endocrine, behavioral, and motor effects explained by clear disturbances of transmitter function, there are other effects:
- Toxic response. Agranulocytosis due to toxic bone marrow depression, particularly with clozapine. Cholestatic jaundice occurs in 2–4% of cases. Skin rashes occur in 5% of patients.
- Ocular problems. Deposits in the cornea and lens occur with chlorpromazine and thioridazine.
- Malignant neuroleptic syndrome. An idiopathic response with fever, extrapyramidal motor disturbance, muscle rigidity, and coma.

Brainstem-acting drugs and general anesthetics

Nausea and vomiting
The vomiting response consists of:
- Reverse peristalsis, where the contents of the duodenum and jejunum are propelled back into the stomach.
- Closure of the glottis.
- Relaxation of the lower esophageal sphincter.
- Contraction of the muscles of the abdominal wall.

These events, together with the sensation of nausea, are coordinated by an area in the medulla. This is known as the vomiting center, which sends its output to the dorsal motor nucleus of cranial nerve X and to the spinal motor neurons innervating the abdominal musculature. The types of stimuli that produce a vomiting response are explained by the inputs to the vomiting center.

The chemoreceptor trigger zone in the area postrema in the medulla senses information about circulating compounds as it is not protected by the blood–brain barrier. Its neural circuits have many receptors (e.g., D_2, $5-HT_3$, opioid) that allow pharmacological intervention to reduce information flow about chemical triggers. Drugs inducing nausea include L-dopa, opioids, anticancer agents (e.g., cisplatin), digitalis, and anesthetics.

The vestibular system sends balance information to the vomiting center. In motion sickness (pallor, sweating, nausea, and vomiting), there is a conflict between the visual and vestibular systems. This can be treated behaviorally or with drugs that reduce vestibular input. Vestibular disease presents with vertigo (false sense of rotary movement), particularly in:
- Labyrinthitis (seen acutely in viral infection, with symptoms of vertigo, nausea, and vomiting).
- Ménière's disease (vertigo, nausea, vomiting, tinnitus, and deafness) produced by increased endolymphatic pressure.

The solitary nucleus sends viscerosensory information about chemicals in the gut collected by cranial nerve X. The enteroendocrine system in the gut wall responds to gut contents and by 5-HT mechanisms can affect the firing of cranial nerve X afferent neurons.

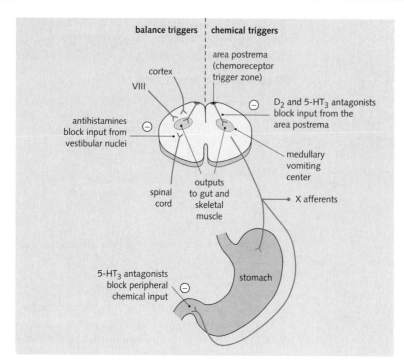

Fig. 13.10 Sites of action of antiemetics.

The spinal cord sends information about trauma: nausea can accompany physical injury.

The limbic cortex sends information from the special senses: certain odors and sights can cause nausea.

Fig. 13.10 summarizes the connections of the medullary vomiting center and the sites of drug action.

Antiemetics

Fig. 13.11 shows the action, uses, and side effects of some antiemetic drugs.

Drugs acting on brainstem monoaminergic systems

The brainstem monoaminergic systems project into the thalamus and cortex with a rather diffuse innervation. This is because these systems have a general modulatory function. Drugs acting on these systems are usually self-administered as drugs of abuse because of their effects on monoaminergic systems that modulate processing of thought and emotion (Fig. 13.12).

General anesthesia

All general anesthetic agents produce:
- Loss of consciousness, of reflex responses to noxious stimuli, of spatial orientation, of volitional

control, and of memory, and reductions in respiratory rate and blood pressure.
- Death at high doses, caused by respiratory depression and cardiovascular depression by actions on the medulla; in addition, cardiac depression may be brought about by direct effects on the myocardium.

Anesthesia used to be characterized by an initial excitatory phase (modern anesthetics act very quickly so that this phase is no longer prolonged or troublesome) followed by a dose-dependent increase in anesthetic depth. This was seen with agents such as ether. Single anesthetic agents are rarely used in modern practice, as their complementary effects allow lower doses to be employed. This leads to fewer side effects. Often a combination of intravenous and inhalational agents is used to exploit their different kinetic properties.

The principles of surgical anesthesia are to produce:
- Loss of consciousness.
- Analgesia.
- Muscle relaxation.

There is no obvious pharmacological structure–activity relationship for anesthetic agents; their mechanisms of action are complex, either by

Antiemetic drugs				
Class	Drug	Site of action	Uses	Side effects
antimuscarinic	hyoscine	vomiting center antagonizing vestibular input	motion sickness	drowsiness, dry mouth, blurred vision, impaired short-term memory
antihistamine	cinnarizine and cyclizine	vomiting center antagonizing vestibular input	motion sickness, vestibular disease	less than antimuscarinics
histamine analog	betahistine	reduces endolymphatic pressure in the membranous labyrinths	Ménière's disease	
D_2 antagonists	metoclopramide and domperidone	chemoreceptor trigger zone reducing sensitivity to chemical triggers in the blood	reduces drug-induced nausea and vomiting; combination with paracetamol to treat migraine	drowsiness, fatigue, motor restlessness
5-HT_3 antagonist	ondansetron and granisetron	chemoreceptor trigger zone and peripherally in the gut reducing transmission from 5-HTergic enteroendocrine cells in response to chemical triggers in the gut	reduces drug-induced nausea and vomiting. Addition of dexamethasone (steroid) increases efficacy in chemotherapy patients requiring high doses	headache, gastrointestinal upset

Fig. 13.11 Antiemetic drugs.

Drug of abuse						
Class	Drug	Action	Effects	Side effects	Tolerance	Dependence
psychomotor stimulants	amphetamine	causes release of NA and DA from terminals	central DA effects: euphoria, excitement, locomotor stimulation with repetitive behavior (stereotypies), anorexia; peripheral NA effects: increased blood pressure, decreased gastrointestinal motility	insomnia, irritability, headache, psychosis, tremor	develops as amphetamine depletes terminals of transmitter	increases activity in DA reward system (VTA to nucleus accumbens), producing psychological dependence
	cocaine	blocks NA and DA uptake (uptake 1)		cardiac dysrhythmias, convulsions, respiratory and vasomotor depression		
hallucinogens	lysergic acid diethylamide (LSD)	5-HT_2 partial agonist	altered perception, thoughts, feelings	persistent effects lasting several weeks, flashbacks to previous "trips"	quickly develops	none
	MDMA (Ecstasy)	amphetamine-like and LSD-like	euphoria and altered thoughts	idiosyncratic responses—coma, convulsions, hyperpyrexia, rhabdomyolysis	cross-tolerance with LSD	none

Fig. 13.12 Drugs of abuse (DA, dopamine; NA, noradrenaline; VTA, ventral tegmental area).

Anesthetic drugs			
Route	Drug	Potency (oil:gas)	Induction/recovery	Notes and side effects
inhaled	N_2O	low (1.4)	fast	Only analgestic by itself. Used 60% O_2/ 40% N_2O as carrier for other agents
	halothane	high (220)	medium	Depresses myocardium, baroreceptor reflex, sympathetic system producing hypotension. 20% metabolized and may cause hepatic damage
	enflurane	medium (98)	medium	Depresses myocardium producing hypotension. 2% metabolized so no hepatic damage. May cause seizures
	isoflurane	medium (91)	medium	Causes vasodilatation producing hypotension. Only 0.2% metabolized. Less epileptogenic than enflurane but may cause myocardial ischemia
injected	thiopentone	high	fast	Depresses myocardium and respiratory center. No analgesic effect. Duration of unconsciousness 5–10 minutes due to liver, kidneys, etc., and then to muscle. Eventual redistribution to body fat so almost total
	propofol		fast	Cardiovascular and respiratory depression. Rapidly metabolized and suitable for total intravenous anesthesia

Fig. 13.13 Anesthetic drugs.

affecting the reticular formation (most anesthetics) or by a direct depression of cortical activity (e.g., propofol).

The potency of any anesthetic is directly related to its hydrophobic nature, generally measured as its lipid solubility as the oil:gas (for gases and vapors) and oil: water (for aqueous agents) partition coefficient. One possible mechanism of action is that anesthetics interact with a hydrophobic region (either lipid, protein, or lipoprotein) of the neuronal membrane, causing membrane expansion and consequent malfunction. Evidence for this is that anesthesia in mammals may be reversed by high ambient pressure (in excess of 100 atm; 10.1 MPa).

Induction and recovery

Induction and recovery describe how quickly anesthesia occurs after administration, and how quickly the body recovers from anesthesia. The speed of induction with, and recovery from, an anesthetic depends upon the physical properties of the anesthetic and how quickly it can equilibrate

between the lungs, blood, and central nervous system for inhalants and gaseous agents, or from blood and central nervous system for aqueous agents.

Intravenous agents (e.g., propofol) are often used for the induction of anesthesia as they can produce unconsciousness in approximately 20 seconds. This is generally preferable for patients as many find facemasks can make them feel claustrophobic.

Inhalational anesthetics (e.g., isoflurane) are more commonly used for the maintenance of anesthesia. This is because they give a more rapid control of the level of consciousness.

After equilibration, 95% of the administered anesthetic is in the body fat. Fat has a low blood flow and so it takes a long time for anesthetics to enter and leave the body fat. A very fat-soluble anesthetic can build up gradually in adipose tissue, and then be released back into the circulation over a long period of time.

The most common general anesthetics are compared in Fig. 13.13.

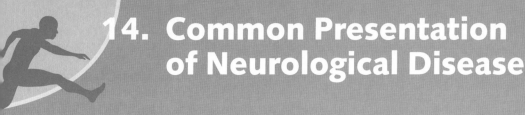
In this chapter, you will learn about:
- Common causes and diagnostic algorithms for common neurological complaints.
- Differential diagnoses are given for:
  - Headache.
  - Central nervous system infection.
  - Dementia.
  - Numbness and tingling.
  - Dizziness.
  - Gait disturbances.
  - Weakness.
  - Coma.
  - Sudden onset of hemiparesis.
  - Seizures.

The most common causes of each complaint are indicated by asterisks. You should consider these first.

Common presenting complaints

Headache
Differential diagnosis (Fig. 14.1)
- Migraine.*
- Tension/stress headache.*
- Chronic daily headache.*
- Cluster headache.
- Hypertension.
- Increased intracranial pressure (ICP) (space-occupying lesion, SOL; cerebral vein thrombosis).
- Infection (meningitis, abscess, postherpetic neuralgia).
- Trauma (head injury, subdural hematoma).
- Vascular (intracerebral hemorrhage, subarachnoid hemorrhage).
- Drug/toxin-related (vasodilators, caffeine withdrawal, carbon monoxide exposure).

Central nervous system infections
Differential diagnosis
This is not strictly a "presenting complaint" but is an important cause of a group of presenting features, as shown in Fig. 14.2.

The list of organisms that may cause central nervous system infection is huge. The most important are listed in Chapter 11.

Dementia
Differential diagnosis
Again, not in itself a "presenting complaint" of the patient, but an important clinical presentation with many underlying causes, as shown in Fig. 14.3.

The surgical sieve, as outlined below, will enable you to remember all the causes of this, but it is more sensible to relate them in an approximate order of likelihood (i.e., think of the asterisked causes first).

Congenital
- Huntington's disease.
- Presenile dementia.
- Adrenoleukodystrophy.
- Canavan's disease.

Acquired
Remember these using the mnemonic "INVITED MD."
- Infective: human immunodeficiency virus, syphilis, Creutzfeldt–Jakob disease, postencephalitis/postmeningitis, progressive multifocal leukoencephalopathy, Whipple's disease.
- Neoplastic: intracranial tumor (benign/malignant, primary/secondary), paraneoplastic.
- Vascular: multi-infarct dementia.*
- Inflammatory: multiple sclerosis.
- Trauma/idiopathic: head injury,* subdural hematoma, normal pressure hydrocephalus, depression.*
- Endocrine: hypo*/hyperthyroidism.
- Degenerative: Alzheimer's disease,* Pick's disease, Parkinson's disease,* Lewy body disease.
- Metabolic: B_{12} deficiency,* see congenital causes, organ failure, anoxia.
- Drugs/toxins: sedatives, chronic alcoholism.

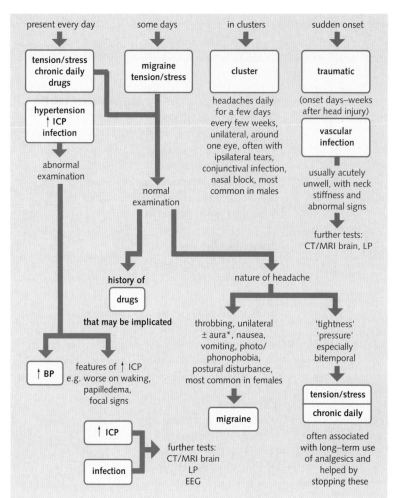

Fig. 14.1 Headache algorithm. *Migrainous auras are transient focal cerebral or brainstem symptoms that accompany the headache (e.g., visual—especially scintillating scotomata; flickering lights in homonomous field) (EEG, electroencephalogram; ICP, intracranial pressure; LP, lumbar puncture).

Numbness and tingling

Differential diagnosis (Fig. 14.4)

Generalized peripheral neuropathy (see Chapter 15). The most common causes are:

- Diabetes:* by far the commonest.
- Vitamin B_{12} and B_1 deficiency.
- Alcohol.
- Carcinomatous.
- Drug-induced.

Isolated mononeuropathy:
- Trauma/compression.
- Mononeuritis multiplex.

Vascular:
- Ischemia (transient ischemic attack, peripheral vascular disease).

Other central nervous system causes:
- Multiple sclerosis.

Anxiety* (particularly fingers and toes).
Idiopathic.*

Dizziness

A very common complaint in neurological practice. Patients may use the term dizziness to describe a wide variety of sensations, including vertigo (a subjective sensation of movement, usually spinning), syncope (faintness and light-headedness caused by decrease in cerebral blood flow), confusion, nausea, headache, numbness, or tiredness. Be aware of this and check what the patient is actually describing.

Most commonly, dizziness describes episodes of either vertigo or syncope. A "funny turn" in

Fig. 14.2 Central nervous system infection algorithm (CXR, chest x-ray; EEG, electroencephalogram; ESR, erythrocyte sedimentation rate; wbc, white blood cells).

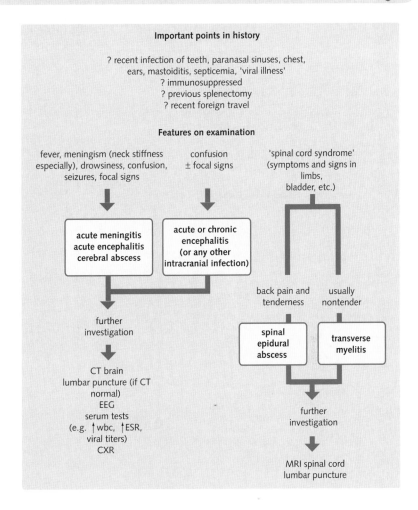

Important points in history

? recent infection of teeth, paranasal sinuses, chest, ears, mastoiditis, septicemia, 'viral illness'
? immunosuppressed
? previous splenectomy
? recent foreign travel

Features on examination

fever, meningism (neck stiffness especially), drowsiness, confusion, seizures, focal signs

confusion ± focal signs

'spinal cord syndrome' (symptoms and signs in limbs, bladder, etc.)

acute meningitis
acute encephalitis
cerebral abscess

acute or chronic encephalitis (or any other intracranial infection)

back pain and tenderness

usually nontender

spinal epidural abscess

transverse myelitis

further investigation

CT brain
lumbar puncture (if CT normal)
EEG
serum tests
(e.g. ↑wbc, ↑ESR, viral titers)
CXR

further investigation

MRI spinal cord
lumbar puncture

neurological practice is usually either one of these or is epileptic in nature.

Differential diagnosis (Fig. 14.5)
Vertigo
Peripheral (inner ear):
- Benign paroxysmal positional vertigo.*
- Benign recurrent vertigo.
- Vestibular neuronitis (also described as peripheral vestibulopathy, or viral labyrinthitis).*
- Ménière's disease.*
- Infection.*
- Head injury.
- Drugs (e.g., aminoglycosides).

Central (in the brainstem or cranial nerve VIII):
- Multiple sclerosis.*
- Brainstem ischemia.
- Basilar migraine.
- Cerebellopontine angle (CPA) tumors.

Syncope
- Simple faint (vasovagal attack).*
- Hypotension, especially postural* (drugs, dehydration, pregnancy, cardiac).
- Transient ischemic attack* (carotid disease, cardioembolism).*
- Cardiac arrhythmia.*
- Syncope induced by micturition, cough, straining, cold foods (ice-cream syncope).

Epilepsy (see Chapter 11)

Gait disturbances
Differential diagnosis (Fig. 14.6)
Weakness
- Upper motor neuron.
- Hemiparesis (stroke,* cerebral tumor, multiple sclerosis), paraparesis (multiple sclerosis,* spinal cord infarction, tumor, cord compression, midline meningioma).

187

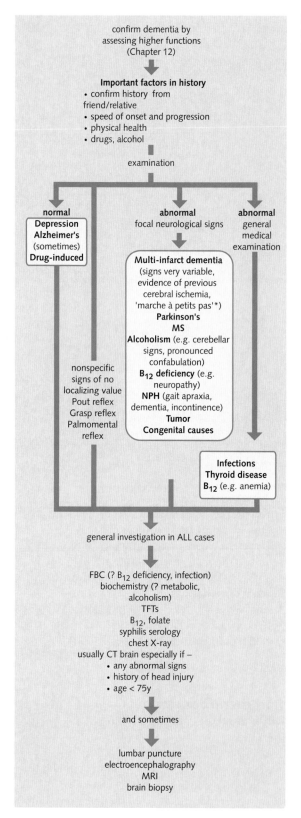

Fig. 14.3 Dementia algorithm. *Describes small-stepped gait typical of (but not specific to) multi-infarct disease (TFTs, thyroid function tests).

Fig. 14.4 Numbness and tingling algorithm (EMG, electromyogram; ESR, erythrocyte sedimentation rate; FBC, full blood count; NCS, nerve conduction studies; TFTs, thyroid function tests).

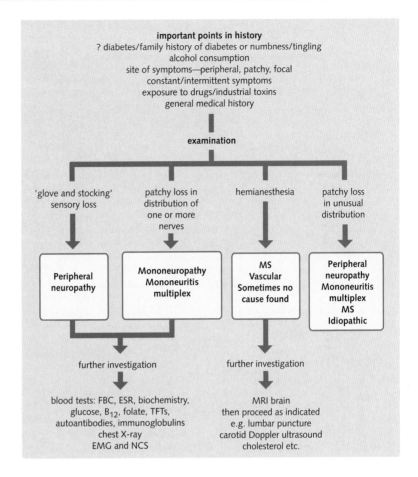

Fig. 14.5 Dizziness algorithm.

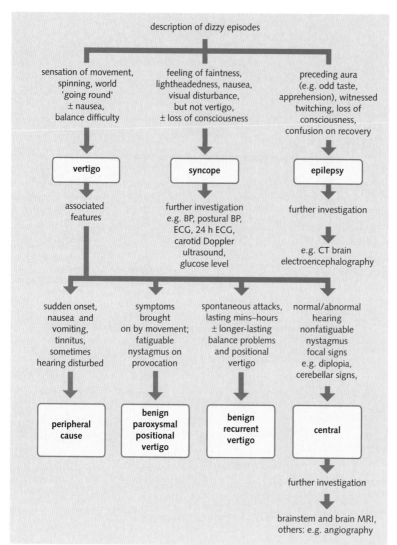

Fig. 14.6 Gait disturbance algorithm (EMG, electromyogram; NCS, nerve conduction studies).

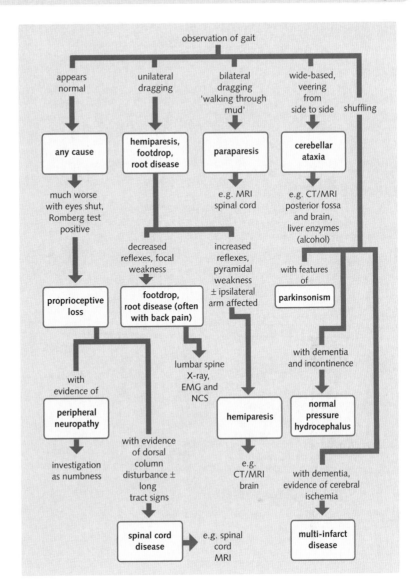

- Lower motor neuron (footdrop,* spinal claudication, root disease).

Ataxia
- Cerebellar disease.
- Proprioceptive loss (peripheral neuropathy).

Extrapyramidal disease
- Parkinson's disease.*
- Other extrapyramidal disorders.

Apraxia
- Normal pressure hydrocephalus.
- Marche à petits pas of multi-infarct disease.

Weakness
Differential diagnosis (Fig. 14.7)
This is best considered from an anatomical point of view, starting at the "top" of the motor tracts and working down. Simple causes are given for each, but you should be able to add to these without difficulty.

Upper motor neuron
- Cortex/cerebral hemispheres (cerebrovascular accident, tumor).
- Brainstem/cerebellar connections (multiple sclerosis, tumor).

191

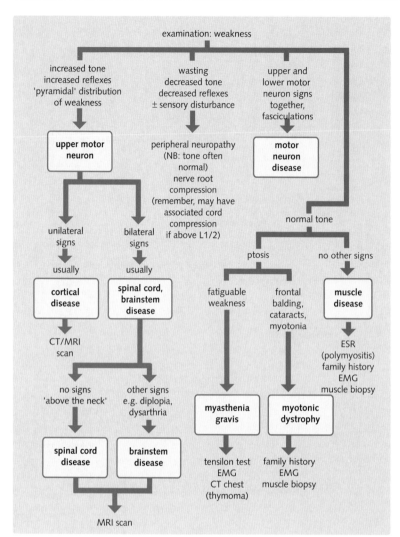

Fig. 14.7 Weakness algorithm (EMG, electromyogram; ESR, erythrocyte sedimentation rate).

- Spinal cord (compression, ischemia, tumor, multiple sclerosis).

Lower motor neuron
- Anterior horn cell (motor neuron disease).
- Nerve root (disk protrusion).
- Peripheral nerve (diabetic neuropathy).

Muscle
- Neuromuscular junction (myasthenia gravis).
- Muscle (muscular dystrophy, polymyositis).

Nonneurological
- Thyroid disorders (hypothyroidism/hyperthyroidism).
- Malnutrition/dehydration.
- Cachexia (underlying carcinoma).

- Electrolyte disturbances (hyponatremia, hypernatremia, hypokalemia, hyperkalemia).
- Pain/stiffness caused by joint disease (arthritis).

Coma
Differential diagnosis (Fig. 14.8)
Intracranial
- Infection* (meningitis, encephalitis, abscess, malaria; see Chapter 11).
- Tumor.
- Cerebrovascular accident* (hemorrhage more commonly than infarction, subarachnoid hemorrhage).

Fig. 14.8 Coma diagnostic algorithm (ABG, arterial blood gases; CVA, cerebrovascular accident; FBC, full blood count; LP, lumbar puncture).

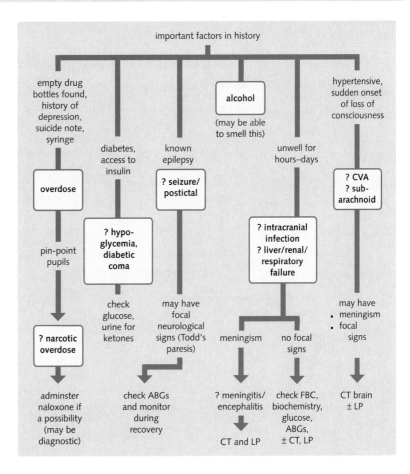

- Anoxic brain injury (following cardiac arrest, head injury, anesthetic accident, respiratory failure).
- Head injury.*

Metabolic
- Hypoglycemia.*
- Diabetic coma* [ketoacidosis, hyperosmolar nonketotic coma (HONK)].
- Liver failure.
- Renal failure.
- Addison's disease, Cushing's disease.
- Hypopituitarism.
- Hyperammonemia (liver failure, amino acid disorders, sodium valproate).

Toxic
- Drug-induced* (including drugs of abuse; heroin, Ecstasy, benzodiazepines and overdose* of most medications).
- Alcohol (excess, Wernicke's encephalopathy).

- Carbon monoxide.
- Hypothermia.

Conditions that may mimic coma
- Akinetic mutism (persistent vegetative state).
- Locked-in syndrome.
- Nonconvulsive status epilepticus.
- Catatonia.

Sudden onset of hemiparesis
Differential diagnosis
Stroke is most likely and may be caused by any of the following:
- Atherothrombotic carotid disease* (predisposing factors—family history, smoking, hypertension, diabetes).
- Cardioembolic disease* (atrial fibrillation, cardiac valve disease).
- Cardiac arrhythmia.*

193

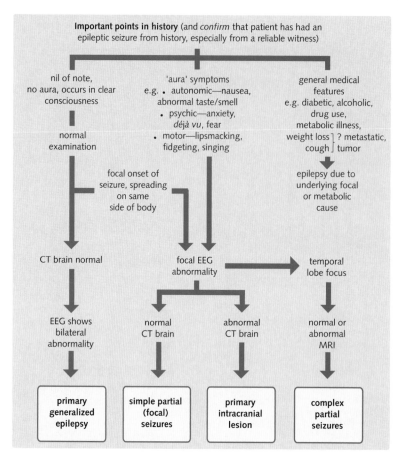

Fig. 14.9 Seizures diagnostic algorithm (EEG, electroencephalogram).

- Hyperviscosity syndrome (multiple myeloma, Waldenström's macroglobulinemia, leukemia).
- Hypotensive episode (watershed infarcts).

However, the differential diagnosis of a patient presenting with sudden collapse with or without focal neurological signs also includes:
- Epilepsy (see also Chapter 11).
- Syncope (see above).
- Most of the causes of coma, especially:
  - Hypoglycemia.
  - Cerebral tumor.
  - Subarachnoid haemorrhage.

Seizures (see Chapter 11)
Differential diagnosis (Fig. 14.9)
- Primary generalized epilepsy.*
- Secondary generalized epilepsy.
- Partial (focal) seizures*:
  - Simple (no impairment of consciousness).
  - Complex (with impairment of consciousness).
- Seizures due to focal structural (tumor, stroke,* infection, trauma) or metabolic (hypoglycemia;* liver failure; drugs,* including overdose; toxins, especially alcohol and alcohol withdrawal*) causes.

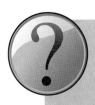

- Outline the important features of the history of a 65-year-old man presenting with confusion.
- How would you approach the management of a 30-year-old woman who complains of a 1-year history of frontal headache?
- A 50-year-old man has been having dizzy spells for a month. What would you do?
- Outline your management of a 20-year-old man who presents to the Emergency Department unconscious.
- How would you distinguish the different types of seizure from history and examination?

15. The Neurological Assessment

In this chapter, you will learn about:
- The observation of a neurological patient.
- Communication skills particularly relevant to patients with neurological problems.
- Examination of the nervous system.
- The examination and assessment of an unconscious patient.

Beginning the interview

Taking a history is the most important part of assessment of the patient with neurological symptoms. Many diagnoses are based on clinical findings alone; the investigations in neurology tend to be expensive and complex, so avoiding them is a bonus.

Observation of the patients as they walk into the examination room or as you approach the bed is vital.
- Do they appear unwell?
- Do they use walking aids (sticks, crutches, frame, wheelchair)?
- Do they appear to be independent, or clearly need help from others?
- Are there any obvious morphological abnormalities (e.g., weakness on one side, drooping of the face, wasting of the muscles)?

As with all examinations, begin your interview by:
- Introducing yourself.
- Explaining who you are.
- Asking if you may talk to and examine them.
- Asking their age and occupation.
- Asking whether they are right- or left-handed.

In the hospital, general observation of the patient's environment is always important.
- Notice the sputum pot and diabetic urine tests.
- Cards and flowers from friends and relatives may indicate a supportive home network.

Immediately, you will observe important points regarding their neurological status.
- Do they respond appropriately (indicating probable preservation of important higher mental functioning)?
- Do they appear to be depressed (which may be part of their neurological condition or may indicate a reaction to it)?
- Do they appear to be elated (again, a feature of some neurological illnesses such as multiple sclerosis)?
- Is their speech normal?
- You may notice additional features such as tremor, agitation, twitches, and abnormal movements. Do not worry about what may be causing these at this stage, as things will become much clearer as you progress through a systematic history-taking process.

The structure of the history

The presenting complaint
From the patient's point of view. Ask:
- "What is the main problem?"
- "What was it that caused you to go to your doctor/come to the hospital?"

When presenting the history to others, use the patient's own words (e.g., "this woman complains of seeing double" rather than "this woman has horizontal diplopia").

The history of the presenting complaint:
- When was it first noted by the patient?
- Has it worsened, improved, or stayed the same since?
- What is its nature (e.g., headache may be sharp, dull, an ache, a throb, etc.)?
- Is there anything that makes it better (e.g., medicines, sleep, exercise) or worse (e.g., time of day, posture, exercise)?
- Have any other symptoms developed since this first complaint was noticed (e.g., main complaint may be weakness of the hand, but a numb patch may have developed more recently)?
- Have any tests already been performed, and if so where and by whom?
- Has the patient ever had other neurological symptoms in the past (these may be related, e.g., an episode of transient visual loss 5 years

previously in a young woman now complaining of difficulty in walking)?
- It is often worth running through a checklist of neurological symptoms.

Neurological symptoms
Remember these by working from the "head down":
- Headache.
- Memory problems.
- Speech difficulty.
- Dizzy turns.
- Swallowing.
- Weakness.
- Numbness.
- Bladder or bowel disturbance.
- Walking difficulty.

Review of systems

Do not underestimate the importance of going through these categories (if only briefly). Coexistent disease may have a huge impact on disability, and may be linked to the presenting complaint (e.g., weight loss and back pain may be indicative of a tumor, which may be related to new-onset neurological symptoms). Things to ask about include:
- Gastrointestinal: appetite, weight loss/gain, swallowing, bowel function (change?).
- Cardiovascular: chest pain, breathlessness, claudication.
- Respiratory: cough, breathlessness.
- Genitourinary: bladder function, impotence, sexual function.
- Musculoskeletal: joint pain, stiffness.

Past medical history

- Any serious illnesses in the past or now? It is useful to write an abbreviated list of important negatives in your examination, to show that these have been checked. The mnemonic "MJTHREADS" is commonly used as a reminder: myocardial infarction, jaundice, tuberculosis, hypertension, rheumatic fever, epilepsy, asthma, diabetes, stroke.

Drug history

- Is the patient taking any medicines now, or have any been taken for some time in the past?
- Are there any known drug allergies?

Family history

- Are there any "family illnesses"? Are parents, siblings, and children alive and well, and if not, what did they die from and at what age? Draw a family tree (Fig. 15.1) if appropriate.

Social history

- Home circumstances: own home, stairs, social-service help, family support, responsibilities for children/disabled relatives, etc.
- Smoking (ever).
- Alcohol (ever heavy consumption).
- Diet (Are they likely to have a vitamin deficiency? Ask about supplementation).
- Heterosexual or homosexual (use your judgment as to whether this is an appropriate question)

Summary

When presenting the history, run through the categories described above, always starting with the same pattern (e.g., "Ms. Randolph is a 40-year-old right-handed administrator who complains of numbness in the feet").

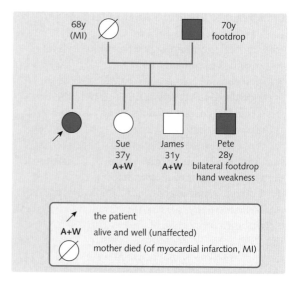

Fig. 15.1 The Lane family tree: an example of autosomal dominant inheritance. In this case, hereditary motor and sensory neuropathy (HMSN).

- Describe the history of the presenting complaint, past medical history, and review of systems. You do not have to mention specifically all negative points, but it is worth pointing out those that are important (e.g., "she has no history of diabetes").
- Say whether the patient is taking any medication.
- Describe the family history, if relevant; if not, explain that "there is no relevant family history."
- Describe important social points (e.g., "she drinks only moderate alcohol and has never smoked").

You will then move on to your examination findings.

When presenting the history, aways start with the same sequence:
- Name.
- Age.
- Handedness.
- Occupation.
- Complaint (in the patient's words).

Communication skills

Patients with neurological problems often present particular problems with communication. This can make them daunting to approach, as we feel embarrassed about our fumblings. Remember that these people have to deal with discrimination and ignorance all the time, and the most important thing you can do is to respect them.

Approaching the patient

Always make sure that you look respectable. Introduce yourself to the patient and ask permission to speak. Always speak to the patient first, rather than any relatives who may be around, even if they appear to be unconscious or incapable of responding. Surprisingly, relatives prefer this too! Many older people like to shake their doctor's hand, but do be aware of cultural differences (see later). Ensure that the patient is comfortable, but that you are too! You don't want to be distracted halfway through the history. Ask the patient's permission to sit on the end of the bed, or to sit on a chair. Preferably you should be at eye level with the patient, or slightly lower. Eye contact is important in building trust with a patient, which you will need when embarking on the examination. It is worth making sure you are in a comfortable position to write.

Beginning the conversation

If possible, leave your note-taking until later—perhaps just jotting down important dates of operations, etc., that you might otherwise forget. Start by checking the patient's name, age, occupation, and handedness. This is a good opportunity to build a relationship—show interest in his occupation, or where he lives. Patients often have fascinating stories to tell, if only people have the time to listen to them!

Begin your history-taking with open questions such as "Tell me what led you to come to hospital" or "Tell me what has been happening with your health lately."

Problems in neurological patients

Be sensitive to any disability that the patient has. If the patient is deaf, make sure you enunciate your words very clearly, and raise your voice if appropriate. Remember that neurological conditions often leave cognitive functions unaffected, so do not speak to any adult patient as if he were a child. Give patients plenty of time, and try not to interrupt—if a patient finds speaking difficult and slow, they probably find it much more frustrating than you do!

Culture and gender

As with all patients, if you are of a different gender, be aware that you may embarrass them by asking them to remove all their clothes. If you need to expose the genital area (or the breasts in females), make it as quick and painless as possible. Cover any part of the patient you are not examining at that moment with a blanket. It is advisable to ask someone of the same sex as the patient to assist you in any intimate examination.

Different cultures approach the gender issue very differently. For example, Muslim women may not feel comfortable shaking the hand of a male doctor. Ask for an assistant if you are in any doubt about how appropriate it is for you to be alone with the patient. This is for your own protection too!

Most patients will not mind you making mistakes with their culture's customs, as long as you apologize and try to learn for the next time. It goes without saying that all cultures should command the same

The neurological examination

Speech

This will probably be one of the first things you assess, albeit unconsciously, during the history.

Speech production is organized at three levels: phonation, articulation, and language production.

Phonation

Phonation is the production of sounds as the air passes through the vocal cords. A disorder of this process is called dysphonia.

Assessment

In dysphonia, the speech volume is reduced and the voice sounds rather husky. Dysphonia is usually due to lesions of the recurrent laryngeal nerves, or to respiratory muscle weakness (e.g., Guillain–Barré syndrome).

Articulation

Articulation is the manipulation of sound as it passes through the upper airways by the palate, the tongue, and the lips to produce phonemes. A disorder of this process is called **dysarthria**.

Assessment

To assess articulation, ask the patient to repeat "baby hippopotamus" and "West Register Street." If the speech articulation is abnormal, this could be caused by:

- Cerebellar dysarthria: speech is slurred (sounds like they are intoxicated), with "staccato" or scanning quality.
- Extrapyramidal dysarthria: speech is soft and monotonous.
- Pseudobulbar dysarthria: speech is high-pitched with a "strangulated" quality and sounds like Donald Duck speech.
- Bulbar dysarthria: speech has a nasal quality that may worsen as the patient continues to speak (suggesting myasthenia gravis).

Language production

Language production is the organization of phonemes into words and sentences, and is controlled by the speech centers in the dominant hemisphere. A disorder of this process is called **dysphasia**.

Assessment

To assess language production:

- Establish the patient's handedness. Dysphasia is a feature of dominant hemisphere dysfunction.
- Listen to the patient's spontaneous speech, assessing its fluency and contents.
- Assess the patient's comprehension by observing his or her response to simple commands: "Open your mouth, look up to the ceiling."
- Assess the patient's ability to name objects. Use your wrist-watch (face, hands, strap, buckle).
- Assess the patient's ability to repeat sentences: "No ifs, ands, or buts."
- If any of these features is abnormal, the patient may be dysphasic (but they must be distinguished from a patient who is depressed and has psychomotor retardation, or severe dysarthria).

Cerebrovascular disease and brain tumors are the most common causes of dysphasia. Dysphasia is classified according to speech fluency and content, comprehension, and anatomical location of the lesions (Figs. 15.2 and 15.3).

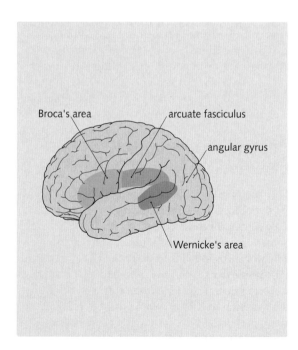

Fig. 15.2 Broca's and Wernicke's areas and their connecting arcuate fasciculus.

Classification of dysphasia					
Type	Lesion	Speech fluency	Speech content	Comprehension of speech	Associations
Expressive	Broca's area	Nonfluent	Normal	Normal	Telegrammatic speech, dysarthria
Receptive	Wernicke's	Fluent	Impaired	Impaired	Neologisms, excessive speech
Conductive	Arcuate fasciculus	Fluent	Normal	Normal	Impaired function in repetitive tasks
Global	Parietal lobe/dominant hemisphere	Nonfluent	Impaired	Impaired	Contralateral visual/sensory inattention, defects in written language, variable extent of other disabilities according to size of lesion

Fig. 15.3 Classification of dysphasia.

Mental state and higher functions
Consciousness
Consciousness is the state of being aware of self and the environment. It has two components:
- The level of arousal.
- The content of consciousness.

The level of arousal
A number of ill-defined terms are used to describe the different levels of arousal:
- Full awakefulness and responsiveness—normal arousal status.
- Obtundation—patient is drowsy and not fully responsive.
- Stupor—patient appears to be asleep, with little or no spontaneous activity; however, he or she is arousable when stimulated.
- Coma—patient is unresponsive and unarousable.

This aspect of consciousness is conventionally assessed using the Glasgow Coma Scale.

The content of consciousness
The content of consciousness is dependent on the patient's level of cognitive functioning. The content of consciousness can be assessed only when a reasonable degree of arousal is present. This aspect of consciousness is conventionally assessed using the mini-mental state examination (see below).

Appearance and behavior
Assessment of the patient's mental state begins as soon as you meet him or her. The physical appearance can be helpful. Demented patients may look bewildered but unconcerned, or apathetic and withdrawn. Look for evidence of self-neglect, which is often concealed by relatives. Observe the patient's response to your questions during the history-taking, assessing his or her comprehension and whether he or she retains insight into his or her problem.

Affect
Ask the patient if he or she has been feeling anxious, depressed, or irritable, and decide if his or her mood is appropriate. Euphoric and manic patients look inappropriately cheerful and energetic, and tend to ignore or play down their problems and disabilities. Patients with emotional lability have sudden unprovoked outbursts of laughing or crying, which can be very distressing to them.

In cognitive impairment, patients' emotional reactions vary according to the severity of their illness:
- At the early stages, anxiety and depression might result from preserved insight into the increasing intellectual difficulties.
- In advanced stages, a flattening of the affect becomes apparent, and may lead to the patient being apparently totally unresponsive.

Attention and orientation
Attention
Ensure that the patient's comprehension is normal. Formal assessment of attention is carried out using serial reversals:

201

- "Can you spell 'world' backwards for me, please."
- "Can you name the months of the year backwards, starting with December."
- "Can you count backwards from 20."

Orientation

Assess the patient's orientation in time, place, and person. To test the patient's orientation in time, ask:

- "What day of the week is it today?"
- "What month are we in?"
- "What time of day is it?"—this is a very sensitive marker for dementia.

To test the patient's orientation in place, ask:

- "Can you tell me where you are now?"
- "What city are we in?"

To test the patient's orientation in person, ask:

- "Who is this person?" (point to a family member, a nurse, or a doctor).

Memory
Immediate memory (recall)

Establish that the patient's comprehension and attention are normal. Immediate recall is tested with digit span: "Can you repeat these numbers after me, please." Start with two or three figures, avoiding recognizable sequences. A normal individual can repeat a five- to seven-digit sequence.

Recent memory

Ask the patient about recent political, social, or sporting events, taking into account his or her premorbid intelligence and socioeconomic status.

Ask the patient to memorize a short address (try "23 West Register Street"). Ask him or her to repeat the address after you to ensure that it has been registered. Distract the patient for the next 10 minutes (by continuing your assessment of his or her mental status), then ask him or her to repeat the address. Most normal individuals will be able to recall all the data in 10 minutes.

Visual memory can be tested by displaying a drawing for 5 seconds and asking the patient to redraw the design 10 seconds later (Fig. 15.4). Patients with visuospatial disorders will have difficulty with the task, even if their visual memory is intact.

Remote memory

Ask the patient about childhood, schooling, work history, or marriage. The accuracy of his or her

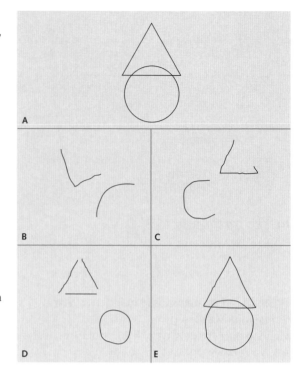

Fig. 15.4 Visual memory test showing (A) the standard design and (B–E) reproductions scored from 0 to 3.

answers should be verified by a relative. If no relative is available, ask a question about a time period relevant to the patient. In elderly people, this might be "In what year did World War Two start?" These questions should again be adjusted for premorbid intelligence and socioeconomic status.

Immediate and recent memory is usually affected early in dementia. However, remote memory is relatively spared in patients with minor degrees of brain damage, but is always affected in those with advanced dementia.

Calculation

This should be tested in the light of the patient's education. Give the patient simple addition or subtraction sums. Serial sevens or threes (subtracting sevens or threes serially from 100) is a useful test.

Dyscalculia is a prominent feature of Gerstmann's syndrome (dyscalculia, right–left disorientation, and finger agnosia), caused by dominant parietal lobe lesions.

Abstract thinking

This is tested by asking the patient to interpret common proverbs:

- "A bird in the hand is worth two in the bush."
- "People in glasshouses should not throw stones."

Abstract thinking can also be tested by assessing the patient's ability to identify the similarities between pairs of objects, e.g., cow and dog, air and water.

Constructional ability and neglect

Constructional ability and neglect are tested by asking the patient to construct simple designs (triangle, square) using matchsticks, and to draw or copy designs of increasing complexity (Fig. 15.5):

- "Please draw a clock, put the hours on it, and set the time at 3 o'clock."

Patients with nondominant parietal lesions have poor constructional ability (which is often associated with neglect to the contralateral side of the body, including the visual fields), which is often reflected in the patients' drawings (they copy only the right side of the design, or they draw and put the numbers on the one side, usually the right side, of the clock).

Right–left disorientation

Establish that the patient's comprehension is normal. Right–left disorientation is assessed by giving the patient simple commands of increasing complexity:

- "Show me your right hand."
- "Put your left hand on your right ear."

Right–left disorientation is seen in patients with dominant parietal lobe lesions.

Apraxia

Apraxia is the inability to perform a skilled movement in the absence of weakness, incoordination, sensory loss, or abnormal comprehension. Apraxia can be confined to the limbs, the trunk, or the buccofacial musculature.

Apraxia is tested by asking the patient to carry out particular tasks of increasing complexity:

- "Stick out your tongue."
- "Pretend to whistle."
- "Show me how to use a toothbrush."
- "Show me how to take the cap off a toothpaste tube and squeeze the toothpaste onto a brush."

There are some special forms of apraxia:

- Dressing apraxia.
- Constructional apraxia.
- Gait apraxia.

Agnosia

Agnosia is the inability to recognize a sensory input in the absence of primary sensory pathway dysfunction. It can affect a certain sensory modality in a global fashion (visual agnosia, auditory agnosia), or it can affect a specific class of stimuli (color agnosia).

Agnosia is tested by showing the patient a few objects and asking him or her to name each one. Allow the patient to manipulate the objects, which might improve recognition (by allowing him or her to use a different sensory input). Assess other sensory modalities:

- Auditory agnosia (inability to recognize sounds).
- Tactile agnosia (inability to recognize objects placed in the hand: astereognosis).
- Finger agnosia (inability to name fingers).
- Topographic agnosia (inability to comprehend three-dimensional sense).

Mini-mental state examination

It is often difficult to perform an extensive testing of higher cortical functions in every patient. Screening tests have been devised to allow rapid assessment. The mini-mental state examination (Fig. 15.6) is one

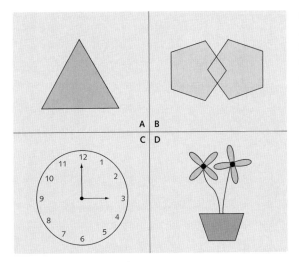

Fig. 15.5 Constructional tests: drawings of increasing complexity to be reproduced by the patient.

Fig. 15.6 The mini-mental state examination.

Mini-mental state examination

Orientation
1. What is the year, season, date, month, day? (one point for each correct answer)
2. Where are we? Country, state, town, hospital, floor? (one point for each answer)

Registration
3. Name three objects, taking 1 second to say each. Then ask the patient all three once you have said them. One point for each correct answer. Repeat the questions until the patient learns all three

Attention and calculation
4. Serial sevens. One point for each correct answer. Stop after five answers. Alternative: spell "world" backwards

Recall
5. Ask for names of three objects asked in question 3. One point for each correct answer

Language
6. Point to a pencil and a watch. Ask the patient to name them for you. One point for each correct answer
7. Ask the patient to repeat "No ifs, ands, or buts." One point
8. Ask the patient to follow a three-stage command: "Take the paper in your right hand: fold the paper in half; put the paper on the floor." Three points
9. Ask the patient to read and obey the following: CLOSE YOUR EYES. (Write this in large letters). One point
10. Ask the patient to write a sentence of his or her own choice. (The sentence must contain a subject and an object and make some sense.) Ignore spelling errors when scoring. One point
11. Ask the patient to copy two intersecting pentagons with equal sides (Fig. 15.5B). Give one point if all the sides and angles are preserved, and if the intersecting sides form a quadrangle

Maximum score = 30 points

Features of cortical and subcortical dementia

	Example	Cognition	Insight	Memory	Response time	Personality	Mood
cortical dementia	Alzheimer's disease, Pick's disease	severely disturbed	absent	difficulty learning new information	normal	unconcerned	may be depressed
subcortical dementia	Parkinson's disease, Huntington's chorea	impaired problem solving	partially retained	difficulty retrieving learned information	slow	apathetic	often depressed

Fig. 15.7 Features of cortical and subcortical dementia.

of many such tests. This is a helpful screening test, but has its limitations.
- The maximum score is 30.
- Scores 28–30 do not support the diagnosis of dementia.
- Scores 25–27 are borderline.
- Scores <25 are suggestive of dementia (if acute confusional state and depression are unlikely).

Cortical and subcortical dementia

Learn to differentiate between the features of cortical and subcortical dementia (Fig. 15.7).

Patients with cortical dementia retain the ability to answer questions at a relatively normal speed. However, their answers are irrelevant and "hopeless."
- Q: How many arms do you have?
- A: Oh, not many!

Patients with subcortical dementia have difficulty in retrieving memories and their response time is therefore long. They are not totally "hopeless" and often find the right answer with some help.
- Q: Who is the current president?
- A: Bill . . . I don't know.
- Q: Is it Bill, Al, or George?
- A: George Bush.

Clinical syndromes associated with specific focal hemispheric dysfunction
Frontal lobe
Conditions associated with frontal lobe dysfunction are:
- Altered personality, altered mood, loss of interest, loss of initiative.
- Expressive dysphasia (dominant hemisphere) and apraxia.
- Hemiparesis and primitive reflexes.
- Sphincter incontinence (bifrontal lesions).

Parietal lobe
Conditions associated with parietal lobe dysfunction on the dominant side are:
- Aphasia, alexia, agraphia.
- Acalculia.
- Right–left disorientation.
- Finger agnosia.

Conditions associated with dysfunction of the nondominant side are:
- Neglect of the contralateral side of the body.
- Constructional and dressing apraxia.
- Topographic agnosia.

Conditions associated with dysfunction of the nondominant or dominant side are:
- Hemisensory disturbance or inattention.
- Lower quadrant homonymous field defect.

Temporal lobe
Conditions associated with temporal lobe dysfunction are:

- Amnesic syndromes.
- Aphasia (dominant lobe).
- Upper quadrant homonymous field defect.

Occipital lobe
Conditions associated with occipital lobe dysfunction are:
- Visual field defects.
- Distortion of vision.
- Impaired visual recognition (visual agnosia).

Gait
In normal gait, the erect moving body is supported by one leg at a time while the other swings forward in preparation for the next support move. Only one foot will be on the floor at any time, although both the heel of the anterior foot and the toes of the posterior foot will be on the ground momentarily when the body weight is transferred from one leg to the other. Normal gait requires input from the motor, sensory, cerebellar, and vestibular systems.

Assessment
The gait of a patient is assessed as follows:
- Ask the patient to walk up and down the examination room in his or her usual fashion, with his or her arms loose by his or her side.
- Observe the patient's posture, the pattern of his or her arm and leg movements, and the control of his or her trunk.
- If gait appears normal, ask the patient to heel–toe walk ("I would like you to walk heel to toe as if you are walking on a tightrope"). Walk alongside the patient to support him or her if he or she appears unsteady.
- If gait appears abnormal, classify it into one of the following patterns:

Hemiplegic gait
Hemiplegic gait (Fig. 15.8A) is caused by unilateral upper motor neuron leg weakness. The arm is held flexed and adducted while the ipsilateral leg is extended (pyramidal pattern of weakness). To move the affected leg, the patient tilts the pelvis to be able to swing the affected leg forward in a "circumduction" manner.

Spastic gait
Spastic gait is caused by bilateral upper motor neuron leg weakness. Both legs are spastic and patients walk in small steps with their toes pressing firmly on the floor as if they are walking in mud. The legs are held

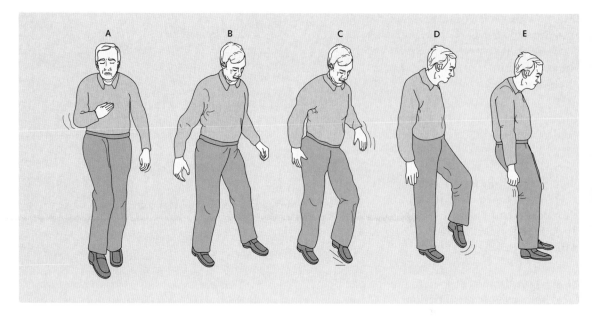

Fig. 15.8 Gait disorders. (A) Hemiplegic, (B) cerebellar ataxia, (C) sensory ataxia, (D) unilateral footdrop, and (E) parkinsonian.

in adduction with the knees touching each other, giving the gait a "scissored" quality.

Cerebellar ataxic gait
Cerebellar ataxic gait (Fig. 15.8B) is caused by cerebellar (and occasionally vestibular) lesions. Patients walk on a wide base and appear unsteady, with erratic body movements. They stagger to the affected side in unilateral lesions (backward if the lesion is in the cerebellar vermis). The condition may be embarrassing for the patient as people assume the patient is drunk. Mild cases can be detected only by asking the patient to walk on a narrow base (heel–toe walking).

Sensory ataxic gait
Sensory ataxic gait (Fig. 15.8C) is caused by proprioceptive and somatosensory loss. The gait is rather unsteady but patients are able to compensate to some extent using their visual input. Patients tend to stamp their feet down against the floor, owing to the loss of all sensory input. Patients become very ataxic in the dark or if the eyes are closed (see Romberg's test).

Footdrop gait
Footdrop gait (Fig. 15.8D) is caused by common peroneal nerve lesion (if unilateral), or peripheral neuropathy (if bilateral). Patients overflex the hip

and the knee to be able to lift their toes off the floor, giving the gait a high-stepping quality.

Parkinsonian gait
Parkinsonian gait (Fig. 15.8E) is slow and shuffling with small stride length, flexed posture, and reduced arm swinging. Patients often have problems in starting to walk and in turning while walking, which is achieved by using an exaggerated number of steps. This gait should be differentiated from the less common *marche à petits pas* seen in bilateral frontal lobe lesions, in which gait is shuffling but the arms and the trunk are not affected.

Waddling gait
Waddling gait is caused by proximal myopathy. Patients have exaggerated lumbar lordosis. They bend their pelvis forward and walk with a waddle, tilting from one side to the other.

Antalgic gait
Antalgic gait is caused by painful musculoskeletal conditions. Patients walk with a "limp" in an attempt to minimize the use of the painful leg.

Apraxic gait
Apraxic gait is caused by parietal lobe lesions. Patients have no difficulty in manipulating their limbs when sitting or lying, but when attempting to

walk they experience great difficulty in organizing their gait and placing their feet in the right positions. Gait appears to have an odd and bizarre character. Patients are liable to "freeze" to the ground, unable to initiate movements.

Hysterical gait

Hysterical gait is erratic and unpredictable. Patients stagger widely with exaggerated arm movements. Falls and injuries are unusual but their presence does not exclude this diagnosis.

Romberg's test

To perform Romberg's test, ask the patient to stand with his or her feet together and assess his or her stability. Next, ask the patient to close his or her eyes, making sure that you will be able to support him or her if he or she falls.

Patients with cerebellar or vestibular lesions are usually ataxic on a narrow base with their eyes open. The ataxia might get marginally worse when the eyes are closed. Patients with proprioceptive sensory loss might be slightly ataxic on a narrow base with their eyes open, but they fall when they close their eyes (positive Romberg's test).

The cranial nerves
Introduction

Examination of the cranial nerves plays an important part in the central nervous system assessment. They provide a number of neurological signs that aid localization, particularly in unconscious patients.

Olfactory nerve (I)

To test the olfactory nerves, first ask patients about any recent change in their sense of smell (anosmia, parosmia, olfactory hallucination) (Fig. 15.9). Then, test their ability to smell coffee, cinnamon, and tobacco, by examining each nostril in turn. Avoid using very irritating odors (e.g., ammonia or camphor), which could stimulate the trigeminal nerve endings, even in anosmic patients.

Unilateral loss of smell is usually asymptomatic. Bilateral loss of smell is usually associated with an altered sense of taste (loss of the ability to appreciate aromas).

Remember to examine the olfactory nerve in all patients presenting with personality changes, disinhibition, or dementia (frontal lobe tumors) and in all cases of head injury.

Causes of olfactory symptoms

Anosmia (loss of smell)
  congenital
  nasal sinuses infections/tumors
  head injury/cranial surgery
  frontal lobe tumors
  subfrontal meningiomas
Parosmia (persistent unpleasant smell)
  nasal infections/tumors
  head injury
  depression
Olfactory hallucination
  temporal lobe epileptic seizures
Paroxysmal, unpleasant smell (burning rubber, smell of gas)
  psychosis

Fig. 15.9 Causes of olfactory symptoms.

The eye (II and III)
Visual acuity (VA)

Visual acuity is tested using a Snellen chart in a well-lit room. Seat or stand the patient 20 feet from the chart. Small, hand-held Snellen charts can be read at a distance of 6 feet.

Near visual acuity is tested using reading charts, but this does not necessarily correlate well with distance acuity.

Correct the patient's refractive errors with glasses or a pinhole. Ask the patient to cover each eye in turn with his or her palm, and find which line of print can be read comfortably. Visual acuity is expressed as the ratio of the distance between the patient and the chart (20 feet) to the number of the smallest visible line on the chart (normally 20/20) (Fig. 15.10).

Color vision

Color vision is tested using Ishahara plates in a daylight-lit room. Test each eye separately. If 13/15 plates or more are read correctly, color vision can be regarded as normal. This test is designed principally to detect congenital color vision defects, but is sensitive in detecting mild degrees of optic nerve dysfunction.

Visual fields

Sit about 3 feet from the patient with your eyes at the same horizontal level. Start by testing for visual inattention. Ask the patient to look into your eyes and hold your hands outstretched halfway between you and the patient. Stimulate the patient's visual

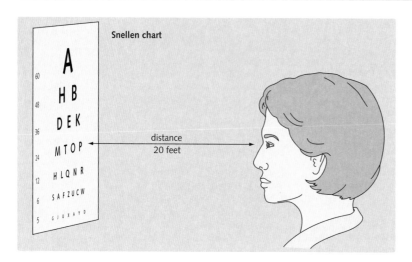

Fig. 15.10 Visual acuity is determined by viewing a Snellen chart at 20 feet.

fields by moving each hand separately and then both hands together, and ask the patient to indicate which of your hands has moved each time.

In patients with parietal lobe lesions, a visual stimulus presented in isolation to the contralateral field is perceived, but it is missed when a comparable stimulus is presented simultaneously to the ipsilateral field (neglect).

Visual fields are examined by confrontation, during which you compare your own visual fields with the patient's (provided that yours are normal). The patient's visual field will match yours only if your head positions are exactly comparable and if your hand is exactly halfway between you and the patient.

Visual fields in poorly cooperative patients are assessed by using visual threat (sudden, unexpected hand movement into the patient's visual field).

Peripheral fields Examine each eye in turn. To test the patient's right visual field, ask him or her to cover his or her left eye with his or her left palm and to look into your left eye throughout the examination.

Cover your own right eye with your right hand, and test the patient's peripheral field by bringing the moving fingers of your left hand into the upper and then the lower quadrants of the patient's temporal fields. Ask the patient to inform you as soon as he or she sees your fingers.

Now cover your own right eye with your left hand and examine the patient's nasal fields with your right hand using the same method.

Blind spot The blind spot is tested using a pen or common lead pencil. Ask the patient to cover his or her left eye and focus on looking at your nose. Move the pen from the central into the temporal field along the horizontal meridian, having explained to him or her that the pen will disappear briefly and then reappear again, and that he or she should indicate when this happens. Once you have found the patient's blind spot, you can map its shape and compare its size with yours.

Central field The central field is tested by moving a pen or pencil along the central visual field (fixation area) in the horizontal meridian. Ask the patient to indicate if the pen tip disappears (absolute central scotoma) or if the color appears diminished (relative scotoma). A central scotoma extends temporally from the fixation area into the blind spot.

Visual field defects Bedside testing of visual fields can detect only large scotomas. Different patterns of visual field defects can be recognized clinically (Fig. 15.11).

Eyelids and pupils

Inspection Note the position of the eyelids. If there is a ptosis, decide whether it is partial or complete; assess its fatigability by asking the patient to sustain upward gaze for at least 1 minute. Next, assess the size and shape of the pupils. They should be circular and symmetrical (Fig. 15.12).

Light response Light responses should be assessed using a bright penlight. Ask the patient to fixate on a distant target and shine the light in each eye in turn from the lateral side. Observe the direct (ipsilateral) and the consensual (contralateral) responses.

Fig. 15.11 Visual field defects (courtesy of Dr. Ross, St. Thomas's Hospital, London).

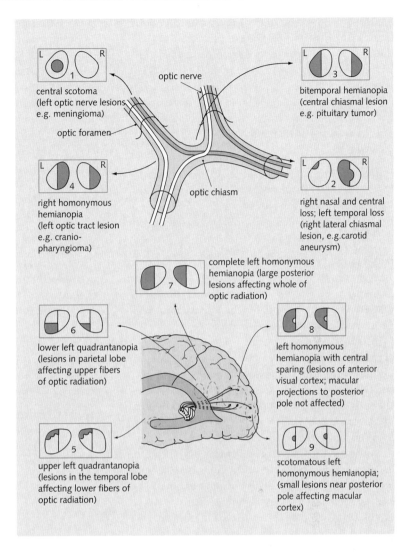

Fig. 15.12 Pupillary abnormalities.

unilateral			reaction to light	associated signs
third nerve palsy			negative	ptosis (partial or complete) external ophthalmoplegia
Horner's syndrome			poor reaction to shade	ptosis (always partial) anhydrosis endophthalmus
Holmes–Adie syndrome			slow reaction	constriction to pilocarpine (0.1%) lower limb areflexia
bilateral				
Argyll Robertson			negative	depigmented iris normal accommodation neurosyphilis
midbrain compression			negative	coma lateralizing signs
pontine stroke			negative	coma hyperventilation hyperpyrexia

Assess the presence of an afferent pupillary defect by swinging the light from one eye to the other, dwelling 3 seconds on each. As you swing the light from, say, the right eye to the left, the pupil of the latter (which has just started to dilate because of loss of its consensual reaction) should immediately constrict. A delayed constriction indicates loss of sensitivity of the afferent pathways (optic nerve damage).

Accommodation　Hold your finger 2–3 feet from the patient and ask him or her to fixate on it. Bring your finger toward the patient's eyes. Observe the normal reaction of bilateral pupillary constriction and convergence (adduction).

Fundoscopy

This is often the most feared part of the neurological examination. The key to picking up signs is simply a matter of practice—try to look at the fundi of every patient you examine.

Ask the patient to fixate on a distant target, avoiding bright lights. Using an ophthalmoscope, examine the patient's right eye using your right eye, and the patient's left eye using your left eye. Warn the patient that you will have to get close to them to do this, and try to keep breathing!

Adjust the ophthalmoscope lens until the retinal vessels are in focus and trace them back to the optic disk. Assess the optik disc shape, color, and clarity of its margins. The temporal disk margins are normally slightly paler than the nasal margins. The physiological cupping varies in size but does not extend to the disk margins.

Next, assess the retinal vessels. The arteries are narrower than the veins and brighter in color. The vessels should not be obscured as they cross the disk margins. Look for retinal vein pulsation, which is present in about 80% of normal individuals and is an index of normal intracranial pressure. This is seen best at the disk margins where the veins cross over the arteries. Note the relative width of the blood vessels.

Assess the remainder of the retina, noting any evidence of discoloration, hemorrhage, or white patches of exudate. Ask the patient to look at the light of the ophthalmoscope, which brings the macula into view. Classify fundoscopic abnormalities into those affecting the optic disk, retinal vessels, or the retina (Fig. 15.13).

Patients with acute optic neuritis might have fundoscopic abnormalities similar to papilledema.

However, in optic neuritis, eye movements can be painful and visual acuity is substantially reduced.

Eye movements (III, IV, and VI)

Inspect the eyes and note the position of the eyelids and the presence of any strabismus (squint). Strabismus is concomitant (usually asymptomatic) if it remains constant throughout the range of eye movements, and incomitant (paralytic) if it varies.

If the patient is capable of voluntary eye movements, the pursuit and saccadic systems should be tested to assess whether eye movements are conjugate, and to detect the presence of diplopia and nystagmus.

Isolated painful third nerve palsy is suggestive of a posterior communicating artery aneurysm.

Pupil-sparing third nerve palsy is suggestive of vascular etiology, particularly diabetes.

Monocular diplopia is suggestive of either refractive defects (cornea or lens) or hysteria.

Very complicated and variable diplopia is suggestive of myasthenia gravis. Look for orbicularis oculi weakness in these cases.

Pursuit eye movements

Steady the patient's head with one hand and hold the index finger of your other hand about 2 feet in front of his or her eyes. Ask the patient to follow your slowly moving finger throughout the range of binocular vision in both the horizontal and the vertical planes in a letter "H" pattern.

Assess the smoothness, speed, and magnitude of the movements. Look for nystagmus, and ask the patient to report any diplopia. In the presence of diplopia, identify the direction of the maximum separation of images and the two muscles responsible for moving the eyes in this direction (Fig. 15.14). Identify the source of the outer image, which comes from the defective eye, by covering each eye in turn. This will allow you to name the muscle(s) and the nerve(s) involved.

Saccadic eye movements

Ask the patient to keep his or her head still, and to look left, right, up, and down as quickly as possible. Assess the velocity and the accuracy of the movements. Look for slow or absent adduction (internuclear ophthalmoplegia) (Fig. 15.15).

If pursuit or saccadic eye movements are absent, oculocephalic reflex (doll's eye movements) will differentiate between supranuclear and nuclear

Fig. 15.13 Common fundoscopic abnormalities.

Structure	Abnormality	Pathology
Common fundoscopic abnormalities		
optic disk	papilledema	raised intracranial pressure, venous obstruction (e.g., cavernous sinus thrombosis, orbital tumor), high CSF protein (e.g., Guillain–Barré syndrome, spinal cord tumors), malignant hypertension, hypercapnia
	optic atrophy	optic neuritis (e.g., multiple sclerosis, Devic's disease), optic nerve/chiasmal compression (e.g., meningioma, optic nerve gliomas, pituitary tumors, Paget's disease of the skull, arachnoiditis), toxic/metabolic (e.g., methyl alcohol, B_{12} deficiency), long-standing raised intracranial pressure), infections (e.g., neurosyphilis), hereditary (e.g., Leber's optic atrophy)
retinal arteries	silver-wiring, increased tortuosity, arteriovenous nipping	hypertension
	gross narrowing with retinal pallor and reddened fovea	central retinal artery occlusion
	cholesterol or platelet emboli	cerebrovascular disease
retinal veins	venous engorgement	papilledema (see above), central retinal vein occlusion
retina	hemorrhages	superficial flamed-shaped (hypertension) and deep dot-shaped (diabetes) subhyaloid between the retina and the vitreous (subarachnoid hemorrhage)
	exudates	soft cotton-wool and hard exudates (diabetes)
	pigmentation	retinitis pigmentosa (e.g., hereditary, Refsum's disease, Kearns–Sayre syndrome), choroidoretinitis (e.g., toxoplasmosis, sarcoidosis, syphilis), post-laser treatment (diabetes)

ocular paralysis. Ask the patient to fixate on your eyes while you rotate his or her head in the horizontal and the vertical planes. In supranuclear lesions the reflex is intact, allowing the patient's eyes to remain fixated on yours.

Ocular nerve paresis

Clinical signs of ocular nerve paresis are shown in Fig. 15.16. Causes of ocular paresis are shown in Fig. 15.17.

Nystagmus

Nystagmus is an involuntary rhythmic oscillation of the eyes caused by lesions affecting brainstem vertical and horizontal gaze centers and their vestibular or cerebellar connections. It is usually asymptomatic, except for oscillopsia when patients experience movements of their visual fields.

Nystagmus must be differentiated from normal endpoint nystagmoid jerks seen at extreme deviation

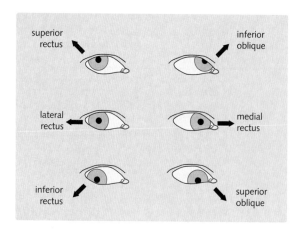

Fig. 15.14 Muscles responsible for eye movements in particular directions.

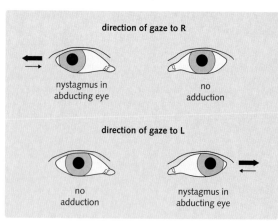

Fig. 15.15 Bilateral internuclear ophthalmoplegia.

Clinical signs of ocular nerve paresis	
Nerve	**Sings**
III	ptosis, eye is deviated laterally and slightly downward (divergent strabismus), pupil may be dilated and unresponsive (pupil staring in diabetes and vascular causes)
IV	impaired depression (and intortion) of the fully adducted eye, head might be tilted to the opposite side to avoid diplopia when reading or looking down
VI	impaired abduction (convergent strabismus)

Fig. 15.16 Clinical signs of ocular nerve paresis.

of gaze, and from the voluntary rapid oscillation of eyes. Both are brief and unsustained.

Testing Note the presence of nystagmus in the primary position of gaze (when looking forward), and while examining eye movements, and decide whether it is pendular or jerky, and whether the movements are horizontal, vertical, rotatory, or of mixed nature.

Record its amplitude (fine, medium, coarse), persistence, and the direction of gaze in which it occurs (the direction of nystagmus is, by convention, the direction of the fast component). Causes of nystagmus are shown in Fig. 15.18.

The face (V and VII)
Trigeminal nerve (V)

Sensory Sensory testing is performed using the same techniques as for the rest of the body

(described later). Test light touch, pinprick, and temperature over the forehead, the medial aspects of the cheeks, and the chin, which correspond to the ophthalmic, maxillary, and mandibular branches of the trigeminal nerve, respectively (Fig. 15.19). A partial loss can be detected by comparing the response to the same stimulus on the other sites on the face.

Corneal response is elicited by lightly touching the cornea (not the conjunctiva) with a wisp of cotton wool. Synchronous blinking of both eyes occurs. An afferent defect (Vth cranial nerve lesion) results in depression or absence of the direct and consensual reflex. An efferent defect (VIIth cranial nerve lesion) results in an impairment or absence of the reflex on the side of the facial weakness. The clinical pattern of sensory loss depends on the anatomical site of the lesion (Fig. 15.20).

212

Fig. 15.17 Causes of ocular paresis.

Causes of ocular paresis		
Type		**Pathology**
supranuclear gaze paresis	horizontal	frontal lobe lesions: eyes deviated to the side of the lesion. Common massive stroke, head injury. Paralysis and voluntary conjugate gaze, with preserved brainstem reflexes (e.g., to coloric stimulation), brainstem pretectal lesions: eyes deviated to opposite side
	vertical	brainstem pretectal region: Parinaud's syndrome (vertical gaze paralysis, papillary dilatation, absent accommodation reflex) extrapyramidal diseases (e.g., Parkinson's disease, progressive supranuclear palsy): impaired vertical gaze (initially upward)
nuclear and nerve (III, IV, VI) palsies	brainstem	vascular lesions, tumors, demyelination, Wernicke's encephalitis
	peripheral	raised intracranial pressure (VI as a false localizing sign, III caused by tentorial herniation) vascular lesions (e.g., atheroma, diabetes, temporal arteritis, syphilis) aneurysms (posterior communicating artery: III, cavernous sinus: III, IV, VI) meningeal inflammation and malignant infiltration skull base tumors (nasopharyngeal carcinoma, chordoma) cranial polyneuropathy (Guillain–Barré syndrome, sarcoidosis) orbital tumors and granulomas, sinus disease
muscle disease		myasthenia gravis, thyroid eye disease, mitochondrial cytopathy

Motor   Inspect for wasting of the temporalis muscles, which produces hollowing above the zygoma. Ask the patient to clench his or her teeth together and palpate the masseters, noting any wasting. The pterygoid muscles are assessed by resisting the patient's attempts to open his or her mouth. In unilateral trigeminal lesions, the lower jaw deviates to the paralytic side as the mouth is opened.

Jaw jerk   Jaw jerk is a brainstem stretch reflex. Ask the patient to open his or her mouth slightly. Rest your index finger on the apex of the jaw and tap it with the patella hammer. The response, mouth opening, is due to a contraction of the pterygoid muscles. An absent reflex is not significant, but the reflex could be brisk in pseudobulbar palsy (see later).

Facial nerve (VII)

Motor response   Inspect the patient's face, looking for asymmetry of the nasolabial folds and the position of the two angles of the mouth. Assess the movements of the upper part of the face by asking the patient to elevate his or her eyebrows, close his or her eyes tightly, and resist your attempt to open them. Movements of the lower side of the face are assessed by asking the patient to blow out his or her cheeks with air, purse his or her lips tightly together and resist your attempt to open them, show his or her teeth, or whistle. Finally, ask the patient to smile, and observe any facial asymmetry.

If you detect any weakness or asymmetry, decide if the weakness is confined to the lower part of the face (upper motor neuron lesion) or both the upper and the lower parts of the face (lower motor neuron lesion) (Figs. 15.21 and 15.22).

Fig. 15.18 Causes of nystagmus.

Causes of nystagmus		
Type	**Description**	**Pathology**
pendular	oscillations of equal velocity	long-standing impaired macular vision (since early childhood), miner's nystagmus
jerky	fast phase toward the side of the lesion	unilateral cerebellar lesions
	fast phase to the opposite side of the lesion	unilateral vestibular lesions
	direction of nystagmus varies with the direction of gaze	brainstem pathology
	upbeat nystagmus	lesions at or around the superior colliculi
	downbeat nystagmus	lesions at or around the foramen magnum
rotatory	specific to one head position, and fatigues with repeated testing	unilateral labyrinthine pathology
rotatory or mixed	all other types	brainstem pathology

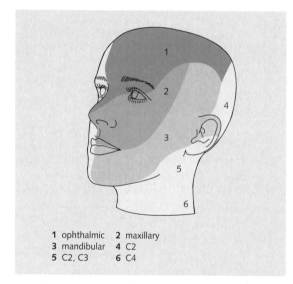

1 ophthalmic   2 maxillary
3 mandibular   4 C2
5 C2, C3   6 C4

Fig. 15.19 Trigeminal sensory innervation to the face.

Do not miss bilateral facial weakness. In this case, the face appears to sag, with lack of facial expression.

Look for Bell's phenomenon (eyeball rotates upward and outward on attempting to close the eye). The lack of this sign may indicate that the patient is not attempting to close his or her eye, raising the suspicion of a psychological reason for the symptoms.

Taste Formal assessment of taste is rarely of practical benefit. Taste is examined by applying a solution of salt, sweet (sugar), or sour (vinegar) to the anterior two-thirds of the tongue and comparing the response on the two sides. The mouth should be rinsed with water between testing. Cranial nerve VIII lesions proximal to the middle ear will cause loss of taste.

Hyperacusis Hyperacusis (undue sensitivity to noise) is suggestive of a lesion proximal to the middle ear, affecting the nerve to the stapedius.

Auditory nerve (VIII)
Hearing
Clinical bedside assessment of hearing is not sensitive, and can detect only gross hearing loss. Audiometry is usually required for detailed assessment. Assess each ear separately while masking the hearing in the other ear by occluding the external meatus with your index finger. Test the patient's hearing sensitivity by whispering numbers into his or her ear and asking him or her to repeat them.

Fig. 15.20 Clinical syndromes of the trigeminal nerve.

Clinical syndromes of the trigeminal nerve		
Site of lesion	**Sings**	**Pathology**
dorsal pons	altered light touch, with preserved pain and temperature.	vascular, tumor
high central medulla	"onion-skin" circumoral analgesia which advances outward	syringobulbia
low central medulla or high intrinsic cervical lesion above C2	"onion-skin" analgesia which starts at the peripheral parts of the face and advances toward the nose and the mouth	syringomyelia
lateral medulla	ipsilateral loss of pain and temperature	lateral medullary syndrome
upper cervical cord, foramen magnum	generalized sensory loss which starts first in ophthalmic division and advances downward	cervical spondylosis, meningiomas
sensory root or ganglia	generalized sensory loss of all modalities	acoustic neuroma, meningioma, angioma
peripheral branch	selective sensory loss of all modalities	orbital tumors, neuromas

Clinical syndromes of facial weakness		
Site of lesion	**Signs**	**Common pathology**
supranuclear	contralateral (or ipsilateral) UMN weakness	vascular, tumor
brainstem	ipsilateral LMN weakness	vascular, tumors, syrinx, demyelination
cerebellopontine	ipsilateral LMN weakness	acoustic neuromas, meningiomas,
angle		angioma
basal meninges	often bilateral LMN weakness	sarcoidosis, malignant meningitis
petrous bone	ipsilateral LMN weakness	middle ear infections, Bell's palsy, geniculate herpetic zoster
face	ipsilateral LMN weakness	parotid tumors, trauma
muscle disease	usually bilateral LMN weakness	myasthenia gravis, myotonic dystrophy, muscular dystrophy
others	usually bilateral LMN weakness	Guillain–Barré syndrome

Fig. 15.21 Clinical syndromes of facial weakness (LMN, lower motor neuron; UMN, upper motor neuron).

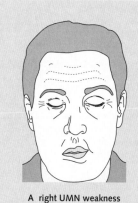
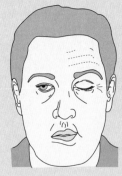
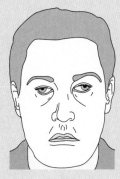

| A right UMN weakness | B right LMN weakness | C bilateral LMN weakness |

Fig. 15.22 Facial weakness. The patient is asked to close his or her eyes and purse his or her lips. Note the defective eye closure and Bell's phenomenon in B and C (LMN, lower motor neuron; UMN, upper motor neuron).

If hearing is impaired, examine the external auditory meatus and the tympanic membrane with an auroscope to exclude infections or wax. Determine if the hearing loss is conductive (middle ear pathology) or perceptive (inner ear pathology) by performing Rinné and Weber's tests.

Rinné test Place a vibrating 512 Hz tuning fork on the mastoid process (bone conduction) and then hold it close to the ear (air conduction). Ask the patient to determine which sound is loudest. Normally, air conduction is louder than bone conduction (positive Rinné). In sensorineural deafness, this will be the same, whereas in conductive deafness, bone conduction will be louder.

Weber's test Place a vibrating 512 Hz tuning fork at the midline over the vertex and ask the patient to determine whether the sound is perceived equally loudly in both ears (normal status), or in one ear more than the other. Sound is heard louder in the affected ear in conductive deafness, and in the unaffected ear in perceptive deafness.

Vestibular functions

Sensory information from the vestibular system is important in the control of posture and eye movements. The vestibular functions are assessed by examining these two areas:

- Posture: patients with vestibular lesions complain of vertigo and are mildly ataxic but usually able to compensate, using their visual input. However, patients with acute vestibular lesions can be markedly ataxic, with a tendency to fall toward the affected side.
- Nystagmus: unilateral vestibular dysfunction causes jerky/rotatory nystagmus with the fast phase toward the unaffected side (see nystagmus).

Hallpike's maneuver Hallpike's maneuver should be performed in all patients with positional vertigo (vertigo precipitated by a particular head position).

Sit the patient at the side of a couch facing away from the edge. Pull the patient quickly backward and to one side so that the head hangs about 30–45° below the horizontal plane rotated to one side (Fig. 15.23). Ask the patient to keep his or her eyes open and to report any vertigo, and look for nystagmus. Sit the patient up and observe any nystagmus. Repeat the maneuver to the other side.

If positive, repeat the maneuver to the same side and determine if the pathology is central or peripheral (not always easy) (Fig. 15.24).

Caloric testing This test is not routinely done in all neurological examinations.

Establish that the patient's tympanic membranes are intact. With the patient lying supine with the head elevated at 30°, flush 250 mL of cold water (30°C) into the external auditory meatus. After a delay of 20 seconds, this produces a tonic deviation of the eyes to the same side with compensatory nystagmus to the opposite side lasting for more than 1 minute. Unconscious patients with intact

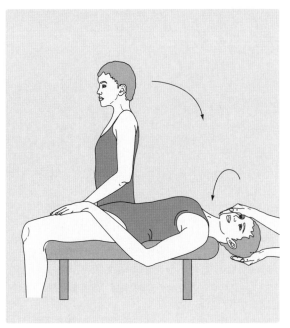

Fig. 15.23 Technique for exhibiting positional nystagmus (Hallpike's maneuver).

Features of peripheral and central positional nystagmus

	Peripheral	Central
site of pathology	semicircular canals	brainstem
vertigo	always present	may be absent
nystagmus	rotatory	horizontal/rotatory
onset	delayed by 3–10 seconds	immediate
repeated testing	response fatigues	usually does not fatigue

Fig. 15.24 Features of peripheral and central positional nystagmus.

Clinical patterns of VIIIth nerve lesions

Site of lesion	Clinical features	Pathology
peripheral	auditory and/or vestibular symptomatology	cranial trauma barotrauma infections occlusion of the internal auditory artery Ménière's disease toxins and drugs
central	auditory or vestibular symptomatology, often with other cranial nerve involvement (V, VII) and long tract signs	cerebrovascular disease multiple sclerosis cerebellopontine angle tumors brainstem tumors syringobulbia

Fig. 15.25 Clinical patterns of VIIIth cranial nerve lesions.

vestibular function will have the tonic deviation only.

The test is repeated 5 minutes later with hot water (44°C), which induces tonic deviation of the eyes to the opposite side and compensatory nystagmus to the side of the irrigated ear.

Labyrinthine or vestibular nerve lesions cause depression of both the "hot" and the "cold" responses from the affected side (canal paresis), whereas central lesions cause an enhancement of nystagmus in one of the directions, whether triggered by hot or cold water (directional preponderance).

Clinical patterns of cranial nerve VIII lesions are shown in Fig. 15.25.

The mouth (IX, X, and XII)
Mouth and tongue
Inspect the tongue as it lies in the floor of the mouth for evidence of wasting (unilateral or bilateral), fasciculations (shimmering movements at the surface

217

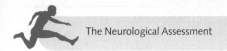
Fig. 15.26 Clinical patterns of tongue weakness.

Clinical patterns of tongue weakness		
lower motor neuron lesions	unilateral	focal atrophy, fasciculations, and deviation to the ipsilateral (paralyzed) side
	bilateral	see bulbar palsy (Fig. 15.27)
upper motor neuron lesions	unilateral bilateral	deviation to the paralyzed side see pseudobulbar palsy (Fig. 15.27)

of the tongue), or other involuntary movements (Huntington's chorea, orofacial dyskinesia). Ask the patient to protrude his or her tongue, and then move it rapidly from side to side. The protruded tongue will deviate to the weak side. If the tongue deviates to one side, it must be examined further for signs of upper or lower motor neuron disease.

Abnormalities can be caused by unilateral or bilateral upper motor neuron or lower motor neuron lesions (Fig. 15.26).

Pharynx and gag reflex

With the patient's mouth wide open, inspect the soft palate, the uvula, and the posterior pharyngeal wall at rest and during phonation (by asking the patient to say "aah").

If you suspect a positive finding (neurological deficit), press the end of an orange stick into the posterior pharyngeal wall, first on one side then the other. Assess the afferent pathway of the gag reflex (IXth cranial nerve) by asking the patient if the sensation is comparable on the two sides, and the efferent pathway (Xth cranial nerve) by inspecting the normal response of a symmetrical rise of the soft palate in the midline. This is a very unpleasant sensation for the patient, and should be carried out with care.

The upper motor neuron innervation of the palatal and pharyngeal muscles is bilateral, and unilateral lesions cause no significant dysfunction. In unilateral lower motor neuron lesions, the palate lies slightly lower on the affected side and deviates to the intact side during phonation or while testing the gag reflex.

Minor and inconsistent deviations of the uvula should be ignored.

The larynx

Formal assessment of the vocal cords is usually performed by indirect laryngoscopy, which is not part of the clinical examination. Bedside evaluation is confined to the assessment of phonation and cough.

Unilateral lesions of the recurrent laryngeal nerve cause partial upper airway obstruction with stridor and hoarseness of voice. Bilateral lesions cause severe stridor and aphonia.

The accessory nerve (XI)

The function of the trapezius muscles is assessed by asking the patient to shrug the shoulders, first without, and then against, resistance. The bulk and the strength of the sternocleidomastoid muscle is assessed by asking the patient to rotate their head to the contralateral side against the resistance of your hand.

Bulbar and pseudobulbar palsies (IX, X, XII)

These syndromes describe bilateral weakness of the bulbar muscles of either an upper or a lower motor neuron type (Fig. 15.27).

Multiple cranial nerve palsies
Patchy loss of function

These palsies are usually caused by:
- Malignant meningitis (due to carcinoma, lymphoma, or leukemia).
- Granulomatous meningitis (due to sarcoidosis, tuberculosis, or syphilis).
- Bone disease (due to metastasis or Paget's disease).

Diffuse loss of function

These palsies are usually caused by:
- Guillain–Barré syndrome.
- Motor neuron disease.
- Myasthenia gravis.
- Polymyositis.

Clinical features and causes of pseudobulbar and bulbar palsies			
	Clinical features	**Cause**	**Pathology**
pseudobulbar palsy	dysarthria (spastic), choking attacks, emotional lability; the tongue is stiff, spastic, slow, but not wasted; jaw jerk and gag reflexes are brisk	bilateral upper motor neuron lesions of IX, X, and XII (supranuclear)	bilateral cerebrovascular disease, motor neuron disease, multiple sclerosis, supranuclear palsy, Creutzfeldt–Jakob disease
bulbar palsy	dysarthria (nasal), dysphagia, and nasal regurgitation; the tongue appears wasted, flaccid, and fasciculating, and the gag reflex is absent	bilateral lower motor neuron lesions	• nuclear: medullary infarction, tumor, syrinx, encephalitis • peripheral nerve: cranial polyneuropathy (e.g., Guillain–Barré syndrome, sarcoidosis, diphtheria), neoplasms (e.g., meningeal infiltration, metastasis), skull base lesions (e.g., metastasis-chordoma, glomus tumor), skull base anomaly (e.g., Chiari malformation) • disorders of neuromuscular transmission: myasthenia gravis • primary muscle disease: polymyositis, muscular, dystrophy

Fig. 15.27 Clinical features and causes of pseudobulbar and bulbar palsies.

Variation in examination findings with site of pathology				
Site of lesion	**Wasting**	**Tone**	**Power**	**Reflexes**
upper motor neuron	none	increased	decreased	increased
lower motor neuron	wasted	decreased	decreased	decreased
neuromuscular junction	rarely	usually normal, decreased	decreased (fatiguable)	usually normal
muscle	sometimes	normal	decreased	decreased

Fig. 15.28 Variation in examination findings with site of pathology. Not every patient will have every feature and occasionally patients may diverge from these features, but this remains a useful guide.

The Motor System
General notes

In most cases, the cardinal sign of motor impairment is weakness. Remember that other findings (signs) will vary with the sites of pathology (Fig. 15.28).

Acute upper motor neuron lesions cause decreased tone (flaccid paralysis) and absent reflexes, although the Babinski response (see below) will be extensor.

Begin, wherever possible, by an inspection of the patient's gait, as outlined earlier. In addition, while the patient is standing:

• Can the patient stand on his or her toes and heels without support?

• Can the patient hop on one leg? (Most patients with significant leg weakness cannot hop.)

Following this, ask the patient to lie on the bed, and make sure his or her arms and legs are exposed.

An examination of the motor system should include the following four features:
• Tone.
• Power.
• Coordination.
• Reflexes.

219

Inspection

When inspecting the patient, look for:

- Wasting—a reduction of muscle bulk in certain muscles compared with others. Wasted muscles are usually weak, and wasting is characteristic of lower motor neuron (i.e., anterior horn cell, nerve root, and nerve) dysfunction.
- Scars—indicating previous injury or surgery, which may have damaged a nerve.
- Fasciculations—seen as rippling or twitching of a muscle at rest, a feature of lower motor neuron problems (especially, but not exclusively, motor neuron disease).
- Involuntary movements such as tremor may be obvious.

Tone

"Tone" means how floppy (decreased tone) or stiff (increased tone) a limb feels. Some patients with increased tone in the legs may complain that their legs "jump," especially in bed.

Some patients have difficulty relaxing during an examination, which can artificially increase stiffness in their limbs. You must therefore do your utmost to put them at ease.

Arms

To examine tone, relax the patient and take his or her arm and slowly flex and extend the elbow, then hold his or her hand, with the elbow flexed, and pronate/supinate the forearm. Try to make your movements as unpredictable as possible, as cooperative patients may unconsciously try to "help" you move their arms. If tone is increased, you may feel a "supinator catch"—an interruption of the smooth movement on supination. Other signs in the arm include cogwheel rigidity, typically seen in Parkinson's disease.

Legs

There are several ways to examine tone in the legs:

- Rock each leg from side to side on the bed, holding it at the knee. Normally, the foot lags behind the leg. If tone is increased, the foot and leg move stiffly, as one unit. If tone is decreased, the foot flops from side to side.
- Flex and extend the knee, supporting both the upper leg and the foot.
- Place your hand under the patient's knee and quickly lift the knee about 6–8 inches. Normally, the foot will stay on the bed; if tone is increased, it may jump up with the lower leg.

Clonus describes the rhythmic contractions evoked by a sudden passive stretch of a muscle, elicited most easily at the ankle. A few beats may be normal in anxious patients, but "sustained clonus" is characteristic of an upper motor neuron lesion.

Increased tone occurs in two main forms:

- Spasticity (derived from the Greek word *spastikos*, to tug or draw) is associated with upper motor neuron lesions, characterized by resistance to the first few degrees of movement, then a sudden lessening of resistance with a "give way" (so-called clasp-knife) effect.
- Rigidity is characteristic of basal ganglia disorders such as Parkinson's disease, distinguished clinically from spasticity by constant resistance (flexion and extension) to passive movement at a joint (lead-pipe rigidity). If tremor is superimposed on rigidity, the resistance is jerky or of "cogwheel" type.

Power

Power needs to be tested in each of the main muscle groups. Power in each muscle is given a grade defined by the following scale (Fig. 15.29), which can initially seem complicated, but is very useful for assessing changes.

The scheme in Figs. 15.30 and 15.31 allows testing of the main muscle groups of the arms. The scheme in Figs. 15.32 and 15.33 allows testing of the main muscle groups of the legs.

Muscle strength	
Grade	Response
0	no movement
1	flicker of muscle when patient tries to move
2	moves, but not against gravity
3	moves against gravity but not against resistance
4	moves against resistance but not to full strength
5	full strength (you cannot overcome the movement with your equivalent muscle group)

Fig. 15.29 The scale for muscle strength.

Fig. 15.30 Testing muscle groups of the upper limb. The blue arrow indicates the direction of movement of the patient, and the black arrow the direction of movement of the examiner.

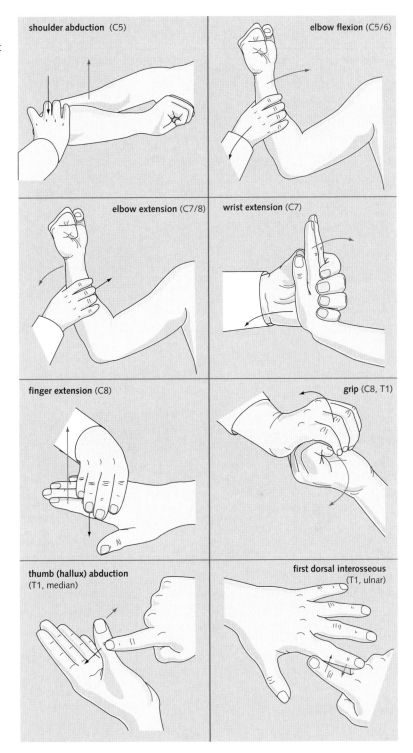

shoulder abduction (C5)

elbow flexion (C5/6)

elbow extension (C7/8)

wrist extension (C7)

finger extension (C8)

grip (C8, T1)

thumb (hallux) abduction (T1, median)

first dorsal interosseous (T1, ulnar)

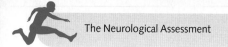
Scheme for examination of power in the upper limbs		
Movement	**Instruction**	**Muscle/myotome**
shoulder abduction	Bend your elbow and hold your arms up and out to the side. Don't let me push them down	deltoid/C5
elbow flexion	Bend your elbow and don't let me straighten it	biceps/C5, C6
elbow extension	Now straighten your elbow and don't let me bend it	triceps/C7, C8
wrist extension	Cock your hands up like this and don't let me stop you	wrist extensors/C7
finger extension	Straighten your fingers out and don't let me push them down	finger extensors/C8
grip	Grip my fingers	finger flexors/C8, T1
thumb abduction	[with palms flat] Point your thumb to the ceiling and don't let me push it down	abductor policis brevis/C8, T1, median nerve
index finger abduction	Spread your fingers wide and don't let me push them together	abductors (dorsal interossei)/T1, ulnar nerve

Fig. 15.31 Scheme for examination of power in the upper limbs. It is useful to get into the habit of giving the same instruction to each patient you examine.

Scheme for examination of power in the lower limbs		
Movement	**Instruction**	**Muscle/myotome**
hip flexion	Lift your leg straight off the bed, keep it up	iliopsoas/L1, L2
hip extension	Straighten your knee and don't let me bend your leg	quadriceps/L3, L4
hip adduction	Keep your knees together and don't let me pull them apart	hip adductors/L2, L3
knee flexion	Bend your knee and keep it bent	hamstrings/L5, S1
ankle dorsiflexion	Pull your foot up toward your nose, don't let me push it down	tibialis anterior and long extensors/L4, L5
plantiflexion (toward the floor)	Point your foot down to the bed, keep it there	gastrocnemius/S1
knee extension	Press your legs flat against the bed and don't let me pull them up	gluteal muscles/L5, S1

Fig. 15.32 Scheme for examination of power in the lower limbs.

Reflexes

Tendon reflexes are most easily determined by briskly stretching the tendon with a reflex hammer, held near the end and briskly tapped either onto the tendon directly or onto a finger placed over the tendon (biceps and supinator) (Fig. 15.34A). You should examine the tendon reflexes in the leg, as shown in Fig. 15.34B. These may be

- Increased.
- Decreased.
- Absent.

Fig. 15.33 Testing muscle groups of the lower limb. The blue arrow indicates the direction of movement of the patient, and the black arrow the direction of movement of the examiner.

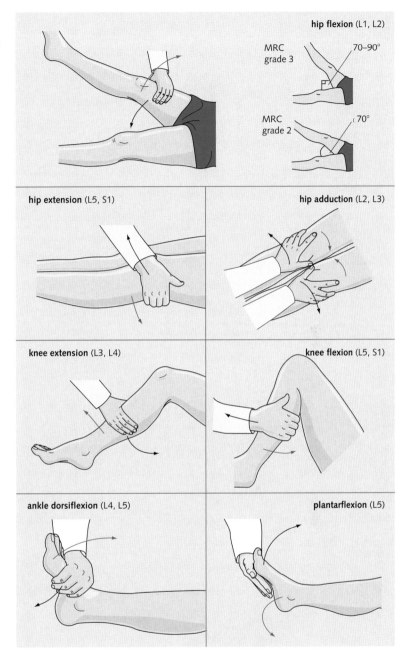

hip flexion (L1, L2)

MRC grade 3   70–90°

MRC grade 2   (70°

hip extension (L5, S1)

hip adduction (L2, L3)

knee extension (L3, L4)

knee flexion (L5, S1)

ankle dorsiflexion (L4, L5)

plantarflexion (L5)

If absent, this should be confirmed by reinforcement (Fig. 15.34C shows this for the legs). There are two methods:

- Asking the patient to clench the teeth tightly just before you tap the reflex.
- Asking the patient to grip the two hands together and pull sideways (hard!) just before you tap the reflex.

The latter is obviously not appropriate when testing arm reflexes.

Tendon reflexes are conventionally graded as shown in Fig. 15.35. Abdominal reflexes can be tested as shown in Fig. 15.34D. The plantar response is elicited by scratching of the sole (Fig. 15.34E).

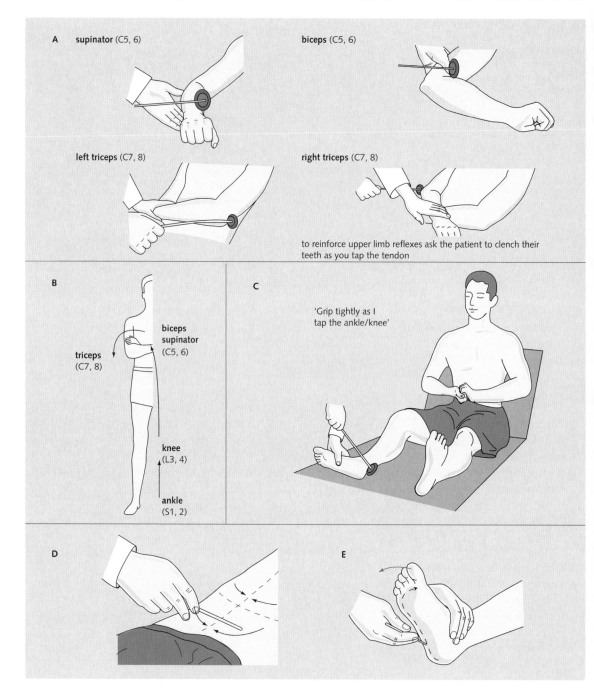

Fig. 15.34 Eliciting reflexes. (A) Upper limb tendon reflexes. (B) A simple way to remember root values of reflexes. (C) Testing ankle jerk with reinforcement. (D) Abdominal reflexes: test in four quadrants shown. (E) The normal response is a downgoing hallux. In an upper motor neuron lesion, the hallux dorsiflexes and the other toes fan out (the Babinski response).

Annotation of tendon reflexes	
normal	+
brisk	++
very brisk, with associated clonus	+++
absent	0
present with reinforcement only (decreased)	±

Fig. 15.35 Annotation of tendon reflexes.

Coordination

Whether a patient can perform smooth and accurate movements is dependent partly on power in the muscles, lack of which may cause clumsiness, but more importantly on the cerebellar system. Assess:
- Gait—a wide-based, sometimes lurching gait is seen in cerebellar disease. Unsteadiness is made more obvious if the patient is asked to walk "heel to toe."
- Arms—the finger–nose test: ask the patient to touch your finger, held about 2 feet in front of the patient, with his or her index finger and then to touch his or her nose, then move back and forth. You may have to move the patient's finger for him or her on the first attempt. Cerebellar lesions may cause "overshooting" of the target, missing your finger (past-pointing) or tremor (intention tremor). Dysdiadochokinesis describes the impairment of rapid alternating movements seen in such patients, and is tested by asking them to slap their palm while alternately pronating and supinating the hand.
- Legs—the heel–shin test: ask the patient to place one heel on the other knee, and slowly slide the heel down the lower leg, then up again. Intention tremor may be seen.

Note that the presence of inaccuracy is the most important sign. These movements must be tested on each side in turn.

Abnormality of these movements in a patient with a cerebellar problem is described as ataxia, and may be associated with other signs of cerebellar disease:
- Nystagmus.
- Dysarthria.

Fine movements

Early stages of an upper motor neuron or basal ganglia disorder may be picked up by noting impairment of fine finger movements: ask the patient to pretend to play a piano, and to touch the thumb with each finger of the same hand in turn.

Abnormal movements (dyskinesias)

Abnormal movements include:
- Decreased movement (e.g., the bradykinesia of Parkinson's disease).
- Increased movement.

The main types of increased movement you will encounter are shown in Fig. 15.36, and may involve the limbs (more usually the arms) and face. All are involuntary.

The most important aspect of examination of dyskinesias is inspection, and most of the features described in Fig. 15.36 can be elicited by this alone. In addition:
- Tremor at rest—ask the patient to sit with his or her hands overhanging his or her lap, close his or her eyes, and count backward from 100 to "bring out" resting tremor.
- Tremor with different actions—the patient will complain if anything in particular makes his or her tremor worse (e.g., holding a cup), so examine those actions in particular. The same applies to myoclonus and dystonias.
- Walking may exaggerate certain movement disorders (e.g., dystonias), so examine this too.

The akinetic rigid syndromes are characterized by abnormal movement:
- Parkinson's disease.
- Steele–Richardson syndrome (with vertical eye movement disturbance and mild dementia).
- Multiple system atrophy:
  - Shy–Drager syndrome (with autonomic failure).
  - Striatonigral degeneration (like Parkinson's but often not responsive to treatment).
  - Olivopontocerebellar atrophy.

When examining a patient with Parkinson's disease, the most commonly encountered disorder of movement, look in particular for:
- Festinant gait—slow, shuffling, flexed, decreased arm swing, unstable on turning, may "freeze." May

Types of abnormal movement (dyskinesia)		
Tremor	**action** physiological drug-induced essential	normal, low amplitude, in outstretched hands exaggeration of normal (e.g., sympathomimetics, lithium) coarser, especially when assuming a posture (e.g., holding a glass); usually autosomal dominant, especially in upper limbs; may involve the head (titubation)
	resting	ask the patient to sit with his hands in his lap, most common in Parkinson's disease
	intention	cerebellar, as above
Jerks	**tic**	abrupt, repetitive, stereotyped jerk-like movements, especially facial; no cause is often found; can be suppressed
	chorea	fleeting, irregular, semipurposeful, disorderly movements affecting any body part; caused by (e.g.) Huntington's disease, stroke involving the subthalamic nucleus (causing ipsilateral chorea, or hemiballismus), drugs (e.g., neuroleptics), or systemic lupus erythematosus
	athetosis	slow, writhing movements, often with chorea
	myoclonus focal segmental generalized	brief, shock-like muscle contractions of one body part (e.g., palatal myoclonus) caused by focal disease of the spinal cord or brainstem and involving body segments supplied by thisregion (e.g., arm) a large number of causes including liver and renal failure, Creutzfeldt-Jakob disease, anoxia, and myoclonic epilepsy May also be *at rest*, with *action* (e.g., postanoxia), or *stimulus sensitive* (e.g., postencephalitis)
Dystonia	**focal** **segmental** **axial** **hemidystonia** **generalized**	sustained muscle contraction causing unusual postures, may be painful involving one body part (e.g., writer's cramp, torticollis) affecting adjacent body segments involving neck and back on one side of the body (e.g., cerebral palsy) all limbs and axial muscles involved (e.g., metabolic disorders—Wilson's disease, Parkinson's disease) drug-induced dystonia may be acute (e.g., metaclopramide, neuroleptics), or chronic (e.g., ʟ-dopa, phenytoin)

Fig. 15.36 Types of abnormal movement (dyskinesia).

show retropulsion (will fall or walk backward if stopped). Initiation of movements is affected, so watch the patient rise from a chair, or start to walk from a stationary position.

- Bradykinesia (slow movements) (especially obvious on fine finger movements).
- Rigidity—carefully examine tone for cogwheeling.
- Tremor—"pill-rolling," at rest.
- Facial akinesia—characteristic absence of facial expression with poverty of movement and lack of expression. May have a "positive glabellar tap": with the hand above the patient, repeatedly tap between the eyes. A normal person will stop blinking after a few taps, but a patient with Parkinson's disease will continue to blink. In practice, this is not particularly useful, but is a favorite with examiners. Increased salivation or drooling may also be evident.
- Handwriting—small and cramped. Keep a sample of this in your examination notes.

Causes of mixed upper and lower motor neuron signs:
- Motor neuron disease.
- Single spinal cord and adjacent root lesion (e.g., cervical spondylosis).
- AIDS.
- Syphilis.
- Chronic upper motor neuron weakness causing "disuse atrophy."

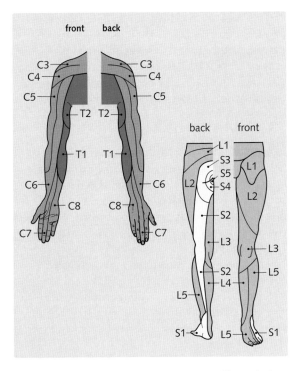

Fig. 15.37 The dermatomes of the upper and lower limbs.

Sensation

General notes
Patients use various terms to describe sensory disturbance, including numbness, weakness, tingling/pins and needles (paresthesia), odd unpleasant touch (dysesthesia), and painful touch (hyperesthesia).

Tell the patient that you are going to test whether he or she can feel certain sensations.

Sensory testing
Do not spend hours doing this, you will exhaust the patient and yourself. Be sensible, and tailor your examination to the patient's complaint.

Remember, sensation from one side of the body travels in sensory tracts to the contralateral cerebral hemisphere.

If the patient complains of loss of sensation, start sensory testing in the abnormal area, and move out from there.

The dermatomes of the upper and lower limbs are shown in Fig. 15.37.

Pinprick
Use a sensory testing/needlework pin, not a needle. Test the pin on the sternum first: "Can you feel this as sharp?" With the patient's eyes open, start at the tips of the fingers/toes and work your way proximally. If the patient does not complain of sensory disturbance, it is not necessary to traverse the entire body with the pin. Remember, this is testing pain sensation. Ask the patient, "Is it sharp or blunt?"

Light touch
Test with cotton wool and with the patient's eyes closed. Start at fingers/toes and work proximally. Ask the patient to "Say yes when you feel me touching you."

Joint position sense
Move the distal interphalangeal joint of the index finger/toe up or down, holding the sides of the digit. With the patient's eyes closed, ask them, "Is your toe/finger moving up . . . or down?" It is useful to demonstrate what you mean by "up" and "down" before testing, as patients often do not understand.

Vibration sense
Use a 128 Hz tuning fork. Set it vibrating, and place it on the patient's sternum. Ask the patient, "Can you feel this vibrating?" Place the tuning fork on the distal interphalangeal joint of the finger or big toe (hallux). Ask, "Can you feel it now?"

Sensation is often lost early in neuropathies.

Two-point discrimination
Test two-point discrimination with specific compasses and with the patient's eyes closed. While testing on the tip of the index finger (normal 3 mm) and hallux (5 mm), ask, "Do you feel one point or two?"

Temperature
With the patient's eyes closed, touch the skin with the flat forks of a tuning fork, not vibrating. Ask, "Does this feel hot or cold?"

Lhermitte's symptom
Lhermitte's symptom is a sudden, electric-shock-like sensation traveling down the neck and back when the neck flexes, caused by a lesion in the spinal cord, most typically multiple sclerosis.

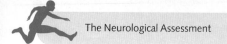

There are five sensations to test.

If the patient complains of sensory disturbance, start testing that area first. If there is no complaint, start distally and move proximally.

Test each sensation in turn in the arms, then each sensation in turn in the legs.

Pain sensation is not agony sensation and therefore do not use a blood-taking needle!

Vibration sense is often lost in neuropathies.

Signs and symptoms of autonomic failure

Affected system or site	Signs and symptoms
cardiovascular system	postural hypotension (or, uncommonly, hypertension); impaired response of pulse to respiration, posture, or Valsalva maneuver resting tachycardia
genitourinary system	impotence, ejaculatory failure, changes in bladder function (including incontinence)
gastrointestinal tract	constipation or diarrhea
secretory systems	inability to sweat; dry mouth and eyes
pupils	Homer's syndrome; dilatation or constriction; sluggish or absent light response

Fig. 15.38 Signs and symptoms of autonomic failure.

The autonomic nervous system

The autonomic nervous system innervates all the viscera, influenced by the hypothalamus via both direct descending pathways and endocrine hormones. It is important to appreciate the anatomy and roles of the individual sympathetic and parasympathetic systems, especially in relation to the effects of drugs on each. However, clinically, "autonomic failure" usually involves both systems simultaneously, most commonly presenting with a combination of symptoms, as shown in Fig. 15.38.

Thorough examination of this system is not necessary in every neurological patient, unless the patient complains of symptoms of autonomic failure or the diagnosis is suspected. The following tests may then be performed at the bedside (more specialized tests may be performed by an autonomic function laboratory).

Examination of the cardiovascular system

Measure the blood pressure after the patient has been lying down for a few minutes. Then stand the patient up, wait for a minute, and take the blood pressure again. The systemic blood pressure normally rises a little. A fall of >20 mmHg is abnormal (postural hypotension).

The pulse can be monitored by a continuous electrocardiogram recording (measurement of the R–R interval is a useful way of measuring such pulse changes) in response to posture, with deep respiration (sinus arrhythmia may be lost) and with the Valsalva maneuver.

The Valsalva maneuver

Ask the patient to take a deep breath in, then blow out through a 20 mL syringe (they will not be able to push the plunger out). Normally, a tachycardia occurs during the forced expiration, followed by a reflex bradycardia on release. The blood pressure drops initially, then is maintained throughout the expiration, before overshooting on release. This response is lost in autonomic failure.

Examination of other systems

The examination of other effects of autonomic failure is more specialized, but includes:
- The pupils (Fig. 15.39).
- Effects of stress (such as grip, arousal, mental activity) on pulse and blood pressure.
- Pharmacological tests of cardiovascular function.
- Sweating responses with heat and pharmacological agents.
- Skin responses to pharmacological agents.
- Urodynamic tests and sphincter electromyography.

Examination of the unconscious patient
Causes of unconsciousness in adults
See differential diagnosis of coma in Chapter 14.

16. Diagnostic Investigations

In this chapter, you will learn about:
- Neurophysiological diagnostic investigations.
- Routine diagnostic investigations (blood tests, etc.) and how they relate to neurological problems.
- Imaging of the nervous system.

Neurophysiological diagnostic investigations

Electroencephalography (EEG)

The EEG measures electrical potentials generated by the neurons lying underneath an electrode on the scalp, and compares this either with a reference electrode or a neighboring electrode. The normal trace is symmetrical, and therefore asymmetries, as well as specific abnormalities, may indicate an underlying disorder. Interpretation of EEGs is complex, and you should not worry if you cannot pick up subtle abnormalities.

Before accurate brain imaging was possible, EEG was used to detect focal lesions. These are now more commonly diagnosed with computed tomography or magnetic resonance imaging, but EEG remains useful for detecting underlying abnormalities of cerebral function, and especially for:
- Epilepsy (see below).
- Diagnosis of encephalitis.
- Coma.
- Aid to diagnosis of Creutzfeldt–Jakob disease.
- Diagnosis of subacute sclerosing panencephalitis.

The main role of EEG is in the assessment of epilepsy. It can help in the following ways:
- Diagnosis of a seizure disorder.
- Classification of seizure type, which may optimize therapy.
- Assessment for surgical intervention.
- Diagnosis of pseudoseizures (especially with simultaneous video recording—telemetry).

Invasive EEG monitoring refers to electrodes inserted directly into the brain. This is undertaken before surgery (e.g., to remove an epileptic focus).

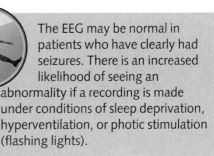

The EEG may be normal in patients who have clearly had seizures. There is an increased likelihood of seeing an abnormality if a recording is made under conditions of sleep deprivation, hyperventilation, or photic stimulation (flashing lights).

Different normal rhythms are characteristically found over different regions of the brain (Fig. 16.1). Other than these rhythmic activities, other abnormal activity may be generated in certain conditions (Figs. 16.2 and 16.3).

Electromyography and nerve conduction studies

Usually performed together, these investigations examine the integrity of muscle, peripheral nerve, and lower motor neurons. They are useful in:
- Determining the cause of weakness (e.g., neuropathy, myopathy, anterior horn cell disease).
- Determining the distribution of the abnormality (e.g., generalized/focal).
- Suggesting the type of myopathy (e.g., dystrophy or myositis) or neuropathy (e.g., axonal or demyelinating; motor, sensory, or sensorimotor).
- Diagnosing myasthenia gravis.
- Assessing baseline deficits before surgery (e.g., carpal tunnel syndrome).
- Objectively assessing the response to medical therapies, especially new treatments in trials (e.g., human immunoglobulin in Guillain–Barré syndrome).

Normal muscle at rest is electrically silent (apart from actually during needle insertion), unless the needle is placed in the region of a motor endplate (when miniature endplate potentials can be recorded). During voluntary movement, individual motor unit potentials (recordings of the activity from the muscle fibers innervated by a single motor neuron) can be seen. Fig. 16.4 shows common abnormalities.

Fig. 16.1 Normal EEG rhythms.

Normal EEG rhythms		
Rhythm	Characteristics	Site and comments
alpha	8–13 Hz (normal)	posterior; especially with eyes closed
beta	>13 Hz (normal)	anterior; increased with sedatives (e.g., barbiturates)
theta	4–7 Hz (normal)	normal in young and when drowsy
delta	<4 Hz (abnormal except in sleep)	slow rhythm generated over a structural lesion and in sleep

Some abnormal EEG activities	
Activity	Interpretation
generalized slow-wave activity	metabolic encephalopathy, drug overdose, encephalitis
focal slow-wave activity	underlying structural lesion
focal/generalized spikes or spike and slow-wave activity	epilepsy
three-per-second (3/s) bilateral. symmetrical spike-and-wave activity (Fig 16.3)	typical absence seizures (idiopathic generalized epilepsy)
periodic complexes (generalized sharp waves every 0.5–2.0 seconds)	CJD

Fig. 16.2 Some abnormal electroencephalographic activities.

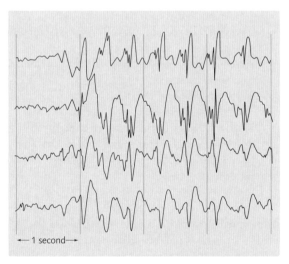

←— 1 second —→

Fig. 16.3 Three-per-second (3/s) spike-and-wave activity. Characteristic of absence seizures.

Fibrillations and fasciculations

Fibrillation potentials (up to 300 mV) are due to spontaneous contractions of individual muscle fibers after denervation, probably due to hypersensitivity of the muscle membrane to acetylcholine. They cannot be seen through the skin, but may be seen in the tongue in motor neuron disease.

Fasciculation potentials (up to 5 mV, usually every 3 or 4 seconds) are contractions of groups of muscle fibers after denervation, visible on both electromyography and through the skin as a twitch or ripple. They may be normal, especially in calf muscles, usually at a rate of 1/s.

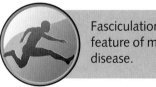

Fasciculations are a particular feature of motor neuron disease.

Fig. 16.4 Common abnormalities found with electromyography (EMG) and nerve conduction studies (NCS) (MUPs, motor unit potenials).

Common abnormalities of the EMG and NCS	
Abnormality	**Change in electromyographic trace**
denervation	Increased insertional activity; large amplitude, long duration, polyphasic MUPs, fibrillations; fasciculations
myopathy	small, short, polyphasic MUPs
myotonia	high-frequency bursts
myasthenia	abnormal decrement on repetitive stimulation; jitter with single-fiber studies (indicating variable neuromuscular transmission time)
Abnormality	**Change in nerve conduction**
axonal neuropathy	small action potential; normal nerve conduction velocity
demyelinating neuropathy	slow nerve conduction velocity; prolonged latency (time to travel from one point to the next); normal or slightly reduced action potential

Other studies

These include:

- Magnetic brain stimulation.
- Evoked potentials (EPs):
  - Visual EPs.
  - Brainstem auditory EPs.
  - Somatosensory EPs.

Routine diagnostic investigations

You should be aware of simple tests of neurological relevance. In this section, five areas of investigation are presented:

- Hematology (Fig. 16.5).
- Biochemistry (Fig. 16.6).
- Immunology (Fig. 16.7).
- Microbiology (Fig. 16.8).
- Cerebrospinal fluid findings (Fig. 16.9).

For each test, normal ranges are given, with neurological differential diagnoses for high and low values. Cerebrospinal fluid protein levels are given in g/dL and serum levels are in g/L.

Imaging of the nervous system

Plain radiography
Skull radiography

Skull radiography has a limited role in current neurological practice. The main indication is head injury when more sophisticated imaging is not immediately indicated. The standard views are:

- Lateral.
- Posteroanterior.
- Towne's view (fronto-occipital).

Learn the normal skull radiographic markings (Figs. 16.10 and 16.11) and the main abnormalities seen on skull radiographs (Fig. 16.12).

Spinal radiography

The standard views in spinal radiography are:

- Lateral.
- Posteroanterior.

Learn the main abnormalities seen on spinal radiographs (Fig. 16.13).

Computed tomography scanning

Using an x-ray source and a series of photon detectors housed in a gantry, computed tomography produces a series of consecutive two-dimensional axial brain digital images, which show the x-ray density of the brain tissue. The densities of different brain tissues vary according to their x-ray absorption properties, ranging between low (black: air, cerebrospinal fluid) to high (white: bone, fresh blood) (Figs. 16.14 and 16.15).

The diagnostic yield of the computed tomography scan is increased by injecting iodine-containing contrast agents, which enhance the distinction

235

Hematology			
Test	Normal range	Abnormality	Possible interpretation
full blood count			
hemoglobin (Hb)	13.5–18.0 g/dL male; 11.5–16.0 g/dL female	low; anemia high; polycythemia	may cause nonspecific neurological symptoms (e.g., dizziness, weakness, fainting); may suggest an underlying chronic illness predisposes to stroke and chorea
mean cell volume (MCV)	76–96 fL	high; macrocytic anemia low; microcytic anemia	vitamin B_{12} deficiency (peripheral neuropathy, SCDC, dementia) may indicate an underlying chronic illness; associated with idiopathic intracranial hypertension
white cell count (WBC)			
neutrophils	$2–7.5 \times 10^9$	high; neutrophilia low; neutropenia	meningitis or other infection leukemia/lymphoma (infiltrative disease, space-occupying lesions, peripheral neuropathy) multiple myeloma (neuropathy, vertebral collapse, hyperviscosity syndrome)
lymphocytes	$1.5–3.5 \times 10^9$	high; lymphocytosis low; lymphopenia	viral infection (transverse myelitis, Guillain–Barré syndrome) leukemia/lymphoma, as above
eosinophils	$0.04–0.44 \times 10^9$	high; eosinophilia	hypereosinophilic syndrome (rare)
platelet count	$150–400 \times 10^9$	high; thrombocythemia low; thrombocytopenia	predisposes to stroke intracranial bleeding
erythrocyte sedimentation rate (ESR)	<20 mm/h	high	vasculitis (e.g., PAN, SLE, giant cell arteritis) may cause cerebral, cranial, and peripheral nerve infarcts, confusion, and seizures)
coagulation tests			
activated partial thromboplastin time (APT or PTTK)	35–45 s	high	SLE; antiphospholipid syndrome
protein C, protein S	varies with laboratory	low; deficiency	inherited predisposition to thrombosis
factor 5 Leiden	varies with laboratory	present	mutation causes a single amino acid substitution in factor 5, which results in activated protein C resistance and predisposition to thrombosis
vitamin B_{12}	>150 ng/L	low; deficiency	peripheral neuropathy, SCDC, confusion/dementia
folate	2.1–2.8 mg/L	low; deficiency	peripheral neuropathy, dementia

Fig. 16.5 Possible consequences of abnormalities in blood or serum levels of hematological indices. Individual laboratories may have different normal ranges (APT, activated partial thromboplastin; PAN, polyarteritis nodosa; PTTK, partial thromboplastin time; SCDC, subacute combined degeneration of the cord; SLE, systemic lupus erythematosus).

Fig. 16.6 Possible consequences of abnormalities in blood or serum levels of biochemical indices. Individual laboratories may have different normal ranges.

Biochemistry			
Test	Normal range	Abnormality	Interpretation
urea and electrolytes (U and Es)			
sodium	135–145 mmol/L	high; hypernatremia low; hyponatremia	both may cause weakness, confusion, and seizures
potassium	3.5–5.5 mmol/L	high; hyperkalemia low; hypokalemia	hyper/hypokalemic periodic paralysis
urea	2.5–6.7 mmol/L	high; renal failure	confusion, peripheral neuropathy
creatinine	<150 mmol/L	high; renal failure	confusion, peripheral neuropathy
glucose (fasting)	4–6 mmol/L	high; diabetes low; hypoglycemia	neuropathy, coma confusion, coma, focal signs
calcium	2.2–2.6 mmol/L	low; hypocalcemia	tetany
liver function tests (LFTs) bilirubin and liver enzymes	bilirubin range: 3–17 µmol/L enzymes vary between laboratories	high	liver disease: confusion, termor, neuropathy
creatine kinase	24–195 U/L	high	muscle disease: myositis, dystrophy
thyroid function tests thyroid-stimulating hormone (TSH)	0.5–5 mU/L	low TSH; thyrotoxicosis high TSH; hypothyroidism	tremor, confusion, hyperreflexia apathy, confusion, hyporeflexia, neuropathy

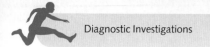

Fig. 16.7 Immunology.

Immunology	
Test	**Associated disorder**
antinuclear factor (ANA)	systemic lupus erythematosus (SLE): seizures, confusion, neuropathy, aseptic meningitis, Sjögren's syndrome: gritty eyes, neuropathies, mixed connective tissue disease (MCTD)
anti-double-stranded DNA (dsDNA) antibodies	SLE
rheumatoid factor	rheumatoid arthritis: cervical spine subluxation, neuropathies, vasculitis
anti-Ro (SSA), anti-La (SSB) antibodies	Sjögren's syndrome
antiphospholipid antibodies (e.g., anticardiolipin)	antiphospholipid syndrome
antiribonucleoprotein (RNP) antibodies	MCTD: myositis, trigeminal nerve palsies
Jo-1 antibodies	polymyositis
antineutrophil cytoplasmic antibodies (ANCA)	pANCA (peripheral): polyarteritis nodosa cANCA (classical): Wegener's granulomatosis
antiacetylcholine receptor antibodies (AChR)	myasthenia gravis
anti-GM1 antibodies	multifocal motor neuropathy, Guillain–Barré syndrome
anti-GAD antibodies	stiff-man syndrome

Microbiology	
Test	**Associated disorder**
VDRL (venereal disease reference laboratory) TPHA (*Treponema pallidum* hemagglutination assay)	primary syphilis; false positive in pregnancy, systemic lupus erythematosus, malaria syphilis; false positive with nonvenereal treponemes (yaws, pinta)
hepatitis B surface antigen (HBsAg)	some cases of polyarteritis nodosa
HIV	AIDS

Fig. 16.8 Microbiology.

Fig. 16.9 Cerebrospinal fluid findings.

CSF findings			
Disease	Protein (g/dL)	Glucose	Cells
normal	<0.5	>50% blood glucose	<5/mL lymphocytes, no polymorphs
bacterial meningitis	1.0–5.0	<50%	>1000/mL, polymorphs predominate
viral meningitis	0.5–1.0	normal	<1000/mL, lymphocytes predominate
tuberculous meningitis	1–10	<50%	<1000/mL, lymphocytes predominate

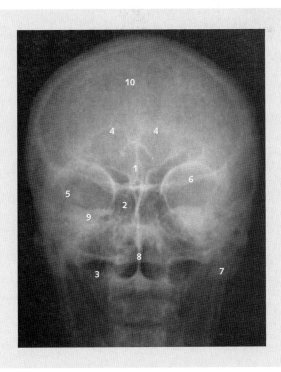

1 crista galli
2 ethmoidal air cells
3 floor of maxillary sinus (antrum)
4 frontal sinus
5 greater wing of sphenoid
6 lesser wing of sphenoid
7 mastoid process
8 nasal septum
9 petrous part of temporal bone
10 sagittal suture

Fig. 16.10 Normal posteroanterior skull radiograph (courtesy of J. Weir and P. H. Abrahams).

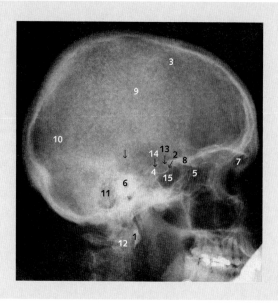

1	anterior arch of atlas (first cervical vertebra)
2	anterior clinoid process
3	coronal suture
4	dorsum sellae
5	ethmoidal air cells
6	external acoustic meatus
7	frontal sinus
8	greater wing of sphenoid
9	grooves for middle meningeal vessels
10	lambdoid suture
11	mastoid air cells
12	odontoid process (dens) of axis (second cervical vertebra)
13	pituitary fossa (sella turcica)
14	posterior clinoid process
15	sphenoidal sinus

Fig. 16.11 Normal lateral skull radiograph (courtesy of J. Weir and P. H. Abrahams).

Main abnormalities seen on skull x-ray	
Pathology	**Abnormality**
trauma	skull fractures, intracerebral hematomas (midline shift of a calcified pineal gland)
tumors	bone erosions (metastasis, multiple myeloma) or hyperostosis (meningiomas), calcifications (craniopharyngioma, glial tumors), enlargement/destruction of the pituitary fossa (pituitary tumors)
raised intracranial pressure	separation of the sutures (children), erosion of the posterior clinoids, thinning of the vault, and flattening of the pituitary fossa
developmental defects	craniostenosis, platybasia
inflammatory processes	opacification of the paranasal sinuses
vascular	calcified intracranial aneurysms and vascular malformations

Fig. 16.12 Main abnormalities seen on skull radiograph.

Main abnormalities seen on spinal x-ray	
Pathology	**Abnormality**
trauma	fractures, fracture–dislocations, subluxations
tumors	erosion of the pedicles (long-standing tumors), erosions of the vertebral bodies (metastatic tumors)
degenerative disease	narrowing of disk spaces, calcification of the intervertebral disks, osteophyte formation

Fig. 16.13 Main abnormalities seen on spinal radiograph.

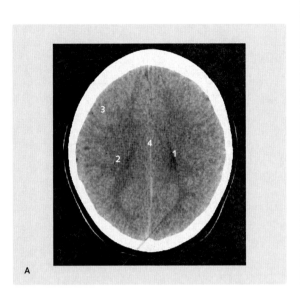

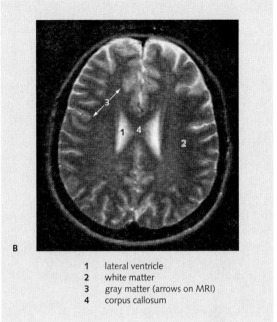

1	lateral ventricle
2	white matter
3	gray matter (arrows on MRI)
4	corpus callosum

Fig. 16.14 (A) Computed tomography and (B) magnetic resonance imaging (T2-weighted image) showing the normal structure of the brain.

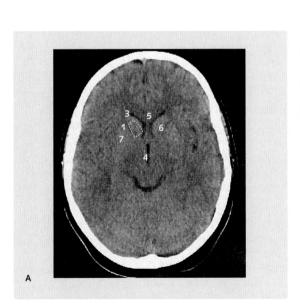

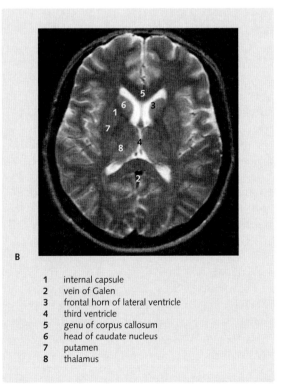

1	internal capsule
2	vein of Galen
3	frontal horn of lateral ventricle
4	third ventricle
5	genu of corpus callosum
6	head of caudate nucleus
7	putamen
8	thalamus

Fig. 16.15 (A) Computed tomography and (B) magnetic resonance imaging (T2-weighted image) showing the normal structure of the brain.

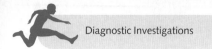
Main abnormalities seen on CT scanning	
Pathlogy	Abnormality
trauma	extracerebral and intracerebral hematomas (HD), brain contusion (mixed HD and LD)
vascular lesions	infarction (LD), hemorrhage (HD), subarachnoid hemorrhage (HD) in the basal cisterns and sulci angiomas, and aneurysms (intensely enhancing lesions)
tumors	enhancing irregular lesions surrounded by LD (edema)
degeneration	brain atrophy (ventricular enlargment, widening of the sulci, and flattening of the gyri)
hydrocephalus	ventricular enlargement whith no evidence of cortical atrophy
infections	abscesses (LD lesions surrounded by ring enhancement), focal encephalitis (LD)
spinal lesions	lesions of the vertebrae, the intervertebral disks, and the spinal canal

Fig. 16.16 Main abnormalities seen on computed tomography scanning (HD, high density; LD, low density).

between the different brain tissues and outline the areas of blood–blood barrier breakdown (around tumors or infarctions). Learn the main abnormalities seen on the computed tomography scan (Fig. 16.16).

Magnetic resonance imaging

Nuclear magnetic resonance is the term that describes the interaction between the hydrogen protons in the different body structures and strong external magnetic fields. As the patient lies in the scanner, the naturally spinning hydrogen protons align with the strong magnetic field of the scanner. When a further external magnetic field (radiofrequency pulse) of a specific frequency is applied at a right angle, the protons "flip" out of the main external magnetic field.

As the protons "relax" back to their original position, they emit a radiofrequency signal that can be digitally analyzed and displayed as an image. This "relaxation" time has two components, known as T1 and T2, which determine the magnetic resonance parameters of the different brain tissues (Figs. 16.14 and 16.15).

The paramagnetic agent gadolinium-labeled DTPA (diethylene triamine penta-acetic acid, or pentetic acid) is used as a contrast agent. Learn the main abnormalities seen on magnetic resonance imaging (Fig. 16.17).

Myelography

A water-soluble iodine-based medium is injected in the subarachnoid space through a lumbar or a cervical approach. This outlines the spinal canal and nerve root sheaths, allowing the assessment of the spinal canal and the nerve roots.

Cord compression caused by extra- or intramedullary lesions is identified as a compression or interruption of the column of contrast.

Postmyelographic computed tomography scanning allows further assessments to the nerve roots within the theca.

Angiography

Serial cranial radiographs are taken after the injection of an iodine-containing contrast agent into a large artery (aorta, carotid, vertebral) to allow the identification of cerebral vessels (Fig. 16.18). Simultaneous digital subtraction of the surrounding soft tissues and bony structures allows the use of more dilute contrast and shorter procedure time, although the spatial resolution of the images will be compromised.

Venous digital subtraction angiography is possible, but the quality of the images obtained is distinctly inferior to those obtained through the arterial route.

The indications for angiography are:
- Extracranial atherosclerotic cerebrovascular disease (stenosis, particularly carotid, lumen irregularities or occlusions).
- Aneurysms and arteriovenous malformation.
- Assessing cerebral vessel anatomy and tumor blood supply before neurosurgery.
- Interventional angiography: embolization of angiomas.

Fig. 16.17 Main abnormalities seen on magnetic resonance imaging.

Main abnormalities seen on MRI	
Pathlogy	**Abnormality**
demyelinating disease	multiple sclerosis (periventricular white malter lesions)
tumors	lesions in the pituitary fossa, cerebellopontine angles, craniocervical junction, and the orbits (images are not affected by artifacts from the surrounding bony structures)
vascular diseases	large aneurysms and venous sinus thrombosis [magnetic resonance angiography (MRA)]
infections	encephalitis, progressive multifocal leukoencephalopathy
spinal lesions	intramedullary lesions (syringomyelia, tumors, demyelination), extramedullary lesions (degenerative disease, tumors, abscesses)

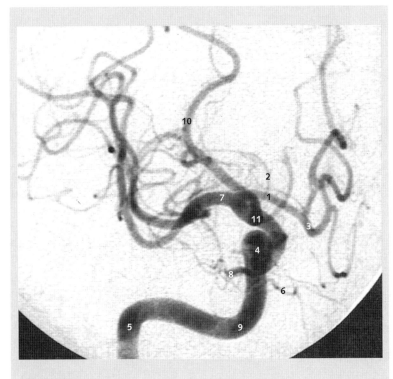

1	anterior cerebral artery
2	anterior choroidal artery
3	anterior communicating artery
4	cavernous portion of internal carotid artery
5	cervical portion of internal carotid artery
6	ethmoidal branch of ophthalmic artery
7	middle cerebral artery
8	ophthalmic artery
9	petrous portion of internal carotid artery
10	posterior cerebral artery
11	posterior communicating artery

Fig. 16.18 Arterial phase of a normal carotid angiogram (courtesy of J. Weir and P. H. Abrahams).

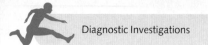

Advantages of magnetic resonance imaging:
- Absence of ionizing radiation.
- The ability to obtain images in coronal and sagittal as well as axial plains.
- More sensitive to the pathological changes in the brain tissues.

Disadvantages:
- Cannot be used for patients with pacemakers (the magnetic field interferes with their function).
- Cannot be used for patients with ferromagnetic intracranial aneurysmal clips or implants (they distort the images and could be displaced by the strong magnetic field).
- Claustrophobia.

Duplex sonography

This technique offers a combination of real-time and Doppler flow ultrasound scanning, allowing a noninvasive assessment of extracranial arteries. It is particularly helpful as a screening test for lesions at the carotid bifurcation which avoids the need for angiography in many patients. The quality of this technique is dependent on the experience and skill of the operator.

Cerebral ultrasonography

This technique is used in neonates, as other imaging requires sedation and/or high radiation doses. The ultrasound is performed through the sutures and fontanelles, which have not fused. It is particularly useful for detecting the presence of hydrocephalus and intraventricular hemorrhage in premature babies.

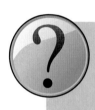

- What rhythms may normally be seen on an EEG? What is the role of the EEG in investigating patients?
- How might you investigate neuromuscular function in someone with myasthenia gravis? How would your findings differ from those in a patient with multiple sclerosis?
- How would you distinguish bacterial and viral meningitis on CSF culture?
- What are the basic differences between computed tomography and magnetic resonance imaging? Give examples of when each is appropriate.
- In what clinical situation might you order a cerebral angiogram? Describe the abnormality you would see.

Index

Page numbers for illustrations are shown in bold type

245

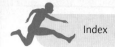

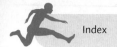

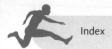

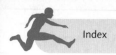

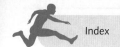

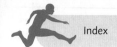

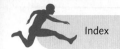